HEALTH-NURSING INFORMATICS & TECHNOLOGY

As per INC

Shivangi Maurya
M.Sc. Nursing
Associate Professor
Sherwood College of Nursing, Barabanki, U.P.

Chirag Giri
M.Sc. Nursing
Assistant Professor
Saraswati College of Nursing, Udaipur, Raj.

Pooran Singh Bhati
M.Sc. Nursing
Assistant Professor
Dakuben Saremalji Sancheti Nursing Institute, Pali, Raj.

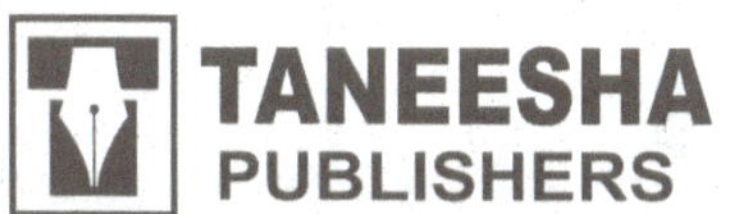

TANEESHA PUBLISHERS

Title   :   Health-Nursing Informatics & Technology

Authors :   Shivangi Maurya, Chirag Giri, Pooran Singh Bhati

Edition   :   First (October, 2024)

ISBN   :   9789348037107

Copyright © 2024, All Rights Reserved by Author

Published by

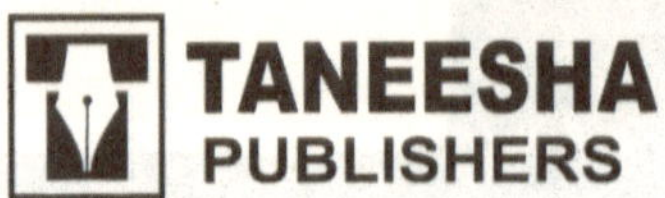

TANEESHA PUBLISHERS | *A Venture by -* PRACHI DIGITAL PUBLICATION

Regd. Add.: 254, Khuriyakhatta No. 10, Bindukhatta, Lalkuan, Nainital - 262402, Uttarakhand, India

Website : www.taneeshapublishers.in

E-mail : taneeshapublishers@gmail.com

Phone : +91 845481 2712, +91 976041 7980

Printed by :

Manipal Technologies Limited, Bengaluru - 560001, Karnataka

COPYRIGHT NOTICE & PUBLISHER DISCLAIMER

Copyright rights of this book including compositions, descriptions, statements, opinions included in this book are reserved by the author, so no any part of this book shall be reproduced partially electronic or mechanical (including film, serial, photographic, without the written permission of the author Recording, any newspaper, magazine, literary portal news portal, blog or translation into another language) in any manner whatsoever without written permission from the author, except in the case of brief quotations embodied in critical articles and reviews. If a person or institution attempts to do so, they will be responsible for the legal action.

Disclaimer : This book has been published with all efforts taken to make the material error-free after the consent of the author. However, the author and the publisher do not assume and hereby disclaim any liability to any party for any loss, damage, or disruption caused by errors Poor omissions, whether such errors or omissions result from negligence, or any other cause. While every effort has been made to avoid any mistake or omission, this publication is being sold on the condition and understanding that neither the author nor the publishers or printers would be liable in any manner to any person by reason of any mistake or omission in this publication or for any action taken or omitted to be taken or advice rendered or accepted on the basis of this work. For any defect in printing or binding, the publisher will be liable only to replace the defective copy by another copy of this book then available through the same seller or distributor where purchased it.

INDEX

Chapter-1

Introduction to Computer Applications for Patient Care Delivery System and Nursing Practice

The usage of computers in healthcare environments is growing. Computer applications can be helpful to nurses in a number of ways. Nurses can receive assistance with patient documentation, scheduling, data analysis, and workflow optimization from computer software and artificial intelligence. Computers are also used for patient communication, treatment documentation, and medication prescription.

Uses of Computers in Teaching Convenience

The life of a student has been greatly facilitated by the use of computers. Students can write and conduct research for their schoolwork online with this device alone. They can also use email or other platforms to connect with teachers and classmates for discussions and knowledge sharing. Undoubtedly, a computer greatly facilitates the life of a student.

Improved Student Performance

It is imperative that computers be used in the classroom as a teaching tool. Students who use computers are more likely to enjoy their studies, which improves performance. When computers are being used, they feel more engaged and concentrated. Furthermore, utilizing computers in the classroom teaches students independence while allowing them to work together.

Fast Access to Research and Information

The days of using the library as the only resource for research and assignment completion are long gone. Accessing all the necessary research materials is now much quicker and easier thanks to computers being used in classrooms. You can find all the solutions you require for your school projects with just a few clicks.

Online Resources

Technology assists students in locating the most accurate and pertinent information when they need assistance selecting a topic for their thesis or essay. The internet and computer technology offer all the most recent information about selecting the ideal thesis topic and the pertinent data to support the choice, regardless of the subject matter—science, business, sociology, or any other course with a name.

Increased Efficiency

Without a doubt, computers help every student be more productive. These enable them to finish their homework, verify their grades, and give presentations even after school. With so much to learn, the efficiency and flexibility that computers offer students make them worthwhile.

Admissions Information

Students can quickly obtain information online when they are attempting to gather as much information as possible about admissions procedures and various universities in order to assist them in selecting which college or university to apply to. Higher education institutions have a very strong internet presence. They can help students with almost anything, including questions about admissions, help with the application and visa processes, payment, and getting ready for arrival. It has benefited students and broadened the scope of universities and other establishments to draw in the top talent from across the globe.

Study Schedules

Technology can assist students in finding the real-time information and updates they need when selecting specific courses. In this manner, students are able to determine the appropriate times for the course; the assignment outlines and aids in helping them plan their study time appropriately.

Better Opportunities

When students use technology and the internet together, they have access to a wide range of opportunities. They can discover comprehensive details about them in this way, determine what best suits their goals and success, and make an informed decision. Through messengers, they can converse with other professionals and gain knowledge from their experiences.

Easy Communication

The use of computers has facilitated communication, particularly for students who reside distant from their families. Even when they are far from home, students can stay in touch with their loved ones through instant messaging, emails, sharing tools, and live updates. In other words, despite distance, the world remains intact thanks to computers and the internet.

Better Rate of Learning

Thanks to technology, a subject that took years to study can now be finished in a matter of hours, particularly in the sciences. These days, software exists that simulates the growth of plants under particular set conditions. The National Library of Medicine/National Institutes of Health of the US government recommends this kind of virtual simulation as an excellent tool for studying growth modeling. Because of virtualization models, it is possible to draw the conclusion that technology helps students learn more in a shorter amount of time.

Visualization Tools

Since many students struggle to visualize the concepts they are taught, math has always been challenging for them. Programs that allow students to view relationships on the computer screen in front of them are now available. Excuse the pun, but they grasp the concept exactly. On the National Library of Virtual Manipulatives, a team from Utah State University has put together a lengthy list of math tools categorized by grade/developmental level. As the data is entered by the students, the chart in front of them is updated. Undoubtedly, abstract concepts are frequently difficult to visualize. With the help of these tools, those ideas become less abstract and more tangible because they are crystal clear and in front of you.

Making Tasks Easier

In place of pricey and bulky textbooks, the majority of schools now provide Chromebooks or tablets. Every subject, workbook, and assignment are available on a small, portable device that weighs no more than two or three pounds and that they can carry with them everywhere they go.

Since they upload each assignment to the Cloud as soon as it is finished, students can no longer use the justifications, "I forgot my assignment in my desk" or "I left my homework at home." All they have to do is select the assignment, go to the relevant file, and log into their student account.

The sole justification is that they left their computer at home, which obviously means that if the school offers internet access, they won't be able to use social media during lunch.

Verdict

There is no doubt that being a student is difficult and stressful. As a student, you have a ton of tasks that you must complete. Because of this, you'll need other technologies, including a computer for school, to get through this stage of your life. Just bear in mind the aforementioned benefits of computers and make sure you select the best one for you. For both current and future generations of students, computers are a great investment.

Uses of Computers in Research

1. **Data collection and analysis:** Researchers use computers to collect, organize and analyze large amounts of data. This includes qualitative and quantitative data, such as surveys, interviews, and experiments.

2. **Simulation and modeling:** Computers can simulate and model complex systems and phenomena, allowing researchers to test hypotheses and predict outcomes. This is particularly useful in fields such as physics, chemistry, and engineering.

3. **Literature review and citation management:** Computers can help researchers to search, organize and analyze academic literature, as well as manage and format citations and references.

4. **Collaboration and communication:** Computers enable researchers to collaborate with colleagues and share their findings with others through various channels, such as online platforms and email.

5. **Visualization and presentation:** Computers can be used to create graphs, charts, and other visual aids to help researchers present their findings in a more effective and understandable way.

Uses of Computers in Nursing

- Electronic Medical Records

- Computerized Scheduling
- Nursing Technology
- Address Issues Easily
- Automated Medication Dispensing
- Computer-Based Patient Care Reporting
- Computer-assisted therapy
- Streamlining workflow
- Data analysis

Electronic Medical Records

Computerized health records that contain data about patients, their ailments, treatment regimens, and advancements are called electronic medical records, or EMRs. Medical professionals, like nurses, can more easily access and share patient data with other medical professionals thanks to electronic medical records (EMRs). Computers can be used to create reports for patients, including diet plans, medication lists, and health status updates, and to store patient data. Computers can be used by nurses to create progress reports for patients and other healthcare professionals.

Computerized Scheduling

Computerized scheduling is used to monitor employee performance and automate the assignment of personnel and resources. In addition, it can be used to find open positions and resolve scheduling conflicts. Computers can be used by nurses to plan their own workloads and monitor the workloads of other nurses and medical personnel.

Computerized scheduling software automatically assigns the right work to the right person by using algorithms to determine the staffing and resources available for a given job. Patient and provider scheduling is automated with the use of scheduling software.

Computers can be used by nurses to plan their own workloads and monitor the workloads of other nurses and medical personnel.

Nursing Technology

Since the 1990s, the use of technology in nursing has grown significantly. During that time, there has been a significant increase in the use of computers in the healthcare industry, as well as in other fields like telemedicine, technology-assisted therapy, and digital health records (DHR). With advancements in healthcare technology, nurses can now fill more positions with greater flexibility. When the nursing staff arrives at a hospital or clinic for a patient appointment, they can use computerized scheduling software to determine which staff members should be assigned tasks.

Electronic medical records (EMRs) are frequently accessible to nursing staff. Patients' medical histories and treatment regimens are kept on file in electronic medical records. Nurse practitioners (NPs) who treat patients in their clinics or hospitals use electronic medical records (EMRs). In order to meet each patient's needs promptly and to provide information about the patient's progress toward treatment goals, they may design personalized electronic medical records (EMRs) for each patient, even if the patient needs diet plans or medication lists.

EMRs can also be used by NPs to schedule tasks and staff positions. It can consider factors like experience, specialization, hours worked, vacation days, and so forth. Computerized scheduling is another tool that nurses can use to help them decide whether to hire more staff.

Address Issues Easily

Computers can be used by nurses to analyze vast amounts of data, including information from diagnostic scans and tests. Patients, other medical professionals, or medical equipment may provide the data. In a healthcare setting, computers can store, sort, and analyze data to find problems or trends. These systems can be used by nurses to recognize and handle problems like possible infections, equipment malfunctions, or patient safety concerns. Nurses can use computer analysis to determine which patients are most vulnerable to a particular result. Additionally, it can assist nurses in determining which patients would benefit from a particular course of care. Nurses can spot patterns with the aid of data analysis, such as which patients are not adhering to their treatment plans or which patients are visiting the emergency room too frequently.

Automated Medication Dispensing

Automated dispensing devices (AMDS) are used by many hospitals to hold and distribute pharmaceuticals. AMDS stores drugs and detects anomalies in the system using computer technology and automated sensors. Medication errors, such as incorrectly identifying a patient's prescription, can be decreased with AMDS. They can assist nurses with medication lists as well. In a medical setting, nurses can order medications and check on their status using computers. Computers, for instance, are able to determine when a patient's prescription is running low and request a refill. In addition, they are able to order replacements for medications that are about to expire.

Computer-Based Patient Care Reporting

Computer-based reporting is a tool that healthcare providers can use to create reports on specific events or patient care. A nurse might, for instance, use a computer to create a report following the administration of a particular kind of medication or the conclusion of a particular treatment. By removing the need for paper documentation, computer-based reporting can save nurses' time. Human error can also be lessened with the aid of computer-based reporting.

Paper jams can cause the reporting process to be slowed down, and paper documentation can raise the possibility of misidentification. Moreover, reports can be produced by computers much more quickly than by paper documentation, often taking only a few seconds.

Computer-assisted therapy

Patients can receive therapy from computers either independently or in combination with other technologies. Computer-assisted therapies include virtual reality therapy, exposure therapy, and cognitive behavioral therapy (CBT).

Stress, depression, and anxiety are among the conditions that computer-based CBT is used to treat. Treatment for specific phobias and anxiety disorders involves exposure therapy. Disorders linked to stress and anxiety can be treated with virtual reality therapy. The advantages of computer-assisted therapy include its affordability and adaptability.

No matter where they are, patients can access the therapy at any time. Apps for smartphones are another way to access some computer therapies. Patients can also choose to finish their therapy in comfort and privacy with computer-assisted therapy.

Streamlining workflow

The use of computer technology can reduce the amount of manual labor required and streamline workflow. Computers can be used by nurses to track workflow, manage tasks, and create reports on staff activities. Multiple task management is possible for nurses with computer-based work management systems.

They can also be used to assign tasks to other staff members, view calendars, and make task lists. These tools can assist nurses in organizing and managing vast volumes of data and assigning tasks according to urgency and importance.

Data analysis

Computer software is a tool that nurses can use to analyze data, including information from diagnostic scans and tests. Patients, other medical professionals, or medical equipment may provide the data. In a healthcare setting, computers can store, sort, and analyze data to find problems or trends.

Nurses can use computer analysis to determine which patients are most vulnerable to a particular result. Additionally, it can assist nurses in determining which patients would benefit from a particular course of care. Nurses can spot patterns with the aid of data analysis, such as which patients are not adhering to their treatment plans or which patients are visiting the emergency room too frequently.

Chapter-2

Principles of Health Informatics

Health Informatics

Information technology is essential to health informatics, also known as health information systems. To enhance patient outcomes, field personnel arrange and review medical records. These employees create protocols for gathering, evaluating, and putting into practice patient solutions utilizing tools and resources already in place. All relevant data about patients, treatments, and potential outcomes must be saved and retrieved. They develop protocols for communication inside the systems of the buildings where they are employed. They guarantee prompt, simple, and effective access to medical records for physicians, nurses, and other professionals. There are numerous degree programs available at every educational level, and the field is expanding quickly.

The network of institutions that collaborate to provide patients with care is made up of businesses, hospitals, and other care facilities. Every facility in this chain needs to be able to speak with every other facility. They need to exchange data securely, swiftly, and accurately. In addition to giving each patient the proper care, the employees, nurses, and physicians must pool their knowledge, experience, and training to advance their methods and procedures. The efficiency and communication between each facility in the care chain are studied by health informatics professionals. Their work is what keeps the quality of care at the highest level and drives process improvement.

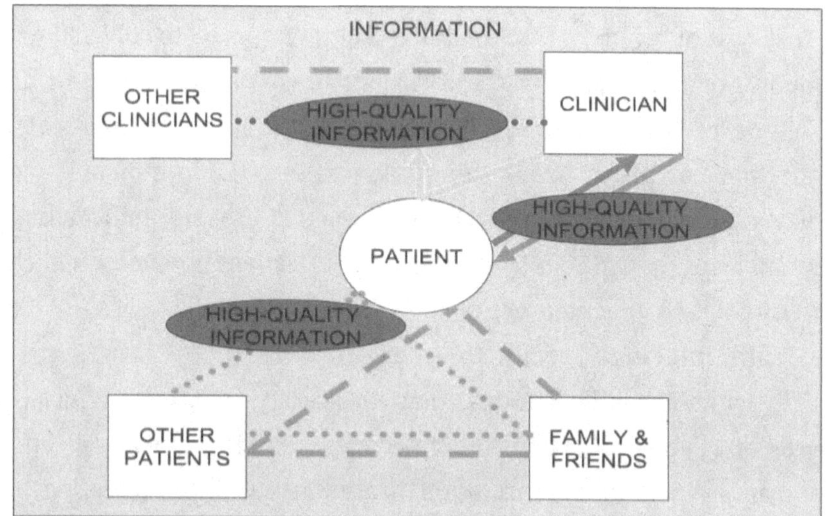

Fig: Concept of Health Informatics

Basic types of health information systems include:

• Transaction processing systems – These types of health information systems process information to complete transactions. Examples of these systems include patient billing systems and hospital admit, discharge and transfer systems.

• Management information systems – These software systems provide management tools for organizing and evaluating departments and/or staff. Examples of information management systems of this type include emergency department and laboratory information systems.

• Decision support systems – These computer systems gather data and uses analytical models and visual tools to improve the outcome of decision-making tasks. The most common examples of this type of system are clinical decision support systems.

Need of Health Informatics

Health informatics reduces healthcare costs

The cost of healthcare is still rising. But the capacity to collect large amounts of data in safe cloud storage has shown to be economical and useful in reducing healthcare expenses. Furthermore, fraud, errors, and financial losses from things like missed appointments and delayed patient care are reduced with the aid of health informatics. The US loses up to $50 billion a year due to patient no-shows, which has a knock-on effect on care quality.

Health informatics reduces error rates

The administrative duties that healthcare workers typically perform, like processing billing codes, filing paperwork, and confirming insurance information, are made easier with the aid of health informatics. By ensuring that patients receive accurate prescriptions based on the data in their medical records, health informatics also helps to minimize medication errors. Care is delivered more effectively and efficiently when these procedures are automated by informaticist-managed quality information systems, which reduces error.

Health informatics improves diagnoses and treatments

The essential component of health informatics is data analytics. Preventive care can be advanced by automated data sorting, which makes it easier for doctors to identify patients who are more likely to have health problems and to treat them before more serious issues arise. A triple benefit of healthcare data analytics is that it can improve care quality, lower medical errors, and expedite communication between insurance companies and healthcare administrators.

Health informatics reduces the length of hospital stays

If a clinician is equipped with the right tools to identify patient risks early on, they can treat patients without needing to stay in the hospital for long. Healthcare providers can obtain up-to-date patient records and medical information through informatics systems, which facilitates crucial decision-making for optimal patient care.

Health informatics empowers patients

Through the use of telehealth services, patients can schedule non-emergency appointments virtually with their primary care physician or specialist, making healthcare delivery simpler, more convenient, and accessible to a larger patient population. During the pandemic, telehealth took off because patients needed to stay in touch with their doctors in order to keep up with regular appointments. This option will continue to help patients with limited mobility, limited access to dependable transportation, or limited access to nearby healthcare facilities now that it has been proven to be an effective medical treatment.

Objectives of Health Informatics

- Developing information systems/processes that improve the quality and efficiency of care
- Building, optimizing, and maintaining electronic health record (EHR) systems
- Designing, developing and evaluating emerging technologies
- Providing data management, analytical, and leadership skills
- Designing and maintaining medical databases, computer networks and applications
- Evaluating the impact of IT on clinical workflow and outcomes
- Developing data analysis and utilization protocols
- Developing privacy and security policies and systems

Limitations of Health Informatics

Expensive

Undoubtedly, the cost of increasingly advanced health technology is high. The aging population is just one of the many issues that all first-world national healthcare systems must contend with. Individuals are living longer. What does this mean, then? As a result, there will be a greater need for healthcare, but fewer people will be working and earning money to support the system.

Requires time to adapt fast

As we all know, technological advancements are ongoing. There will frequently be new software, updates, and methods of operation. Hospital workers need to stay up to date with these developments in order to maintain a competitive edge. Some people may find this difficult, especially the more senior employees.

Over-dependency on technology

The next issue arises after the staff has adjusted to the new work style. Technical problems with computer systems are not unusual. This also applies to the health care informatics system. This is a particularly important issue for the Accident and Emergency (A&E) Department. The hospital's departments are linked together by a shared information system. Several departments are impacted when one is unavailable. One patient, for instance, was hurried into the A&E unit. The subsequent procedures will be delayed if there is an error when retrieving blood analysis information. This will be extremely inconvenient, or worse, it might even negatively impact the patient's health.

Susceptibility to network hackers

For moral and legal reasons, patient medical records and other health information should be kept private. Although the network of the health care system is undoubtedly protected by security measures, network hacking is still a possibility. Thus, there is no doubt that this is a weakness in health informatics.

❖ **Use of Data, Information and Knowledge for More Effective**

Healthcare and Better Health

The ability to coordinate service delivery across the provider network and prevent service duplication is necessary for an effective, integrated health services delivery enterprise. It must be able to link patients and pertinent clinical data regardless of the type of facility that provided the services. Gathering, organizing, and deriving value from data gathered during the delivery of healthcare present many difficulties.

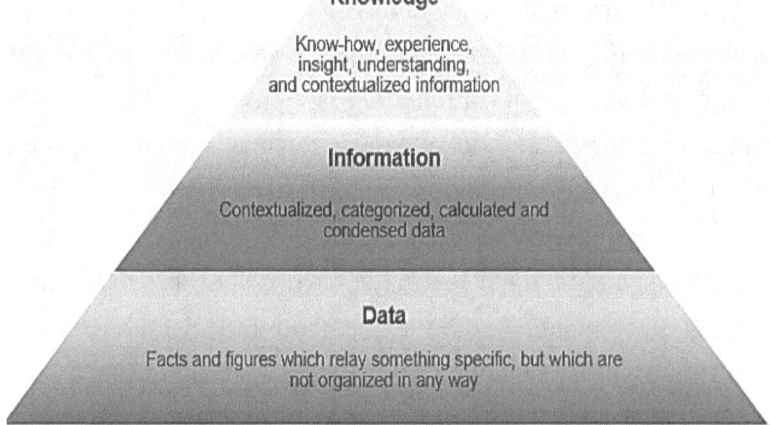

Fig: Relationship between Data, information & Knowledge

Data, Information & Knowledge

Information systems store data, which are the basic building block of cognition and the universal basis for all constructs. Information and knowledge are derived from data and are situated along a continuum that ultimately leads to wisdom. Facts and specified characteristics, like name, gender, date of birth, address, phone number, temperature, and so on, are considered data. Data become semantic data, or information, when meaning is applied to them. The next level of knowledge involves contextualized information, or information that has been interpreted by and from the viewpoint of the recipient. On this continuum, wisdom is the highest level, denoting a state of refined, sublimated knowledge that enables the recipient to maximize interaction with the surroundings.

From Data to Information and Knowledge

In many instances the distinction between information and knowledge is rather ambiguous. Certain users may interpret one set of data as information, while for others it is knowledge.

An information system stores data and metadata—data about data—in a database to reduce ambiguity. Information is created and interpreted with the aid of metadata. The same data is frequently stored by large organizations across multiple systems. When attempting to interpret data, one must consider metadata specific to each system. Before information can be derived from data, sometimes additional data elements must be taken into consideration together (for instance, a patient's name may be stored in three different data fields, as first name, middle name, and last name). Healthcare organizations face considerable challenges when trying to access patient data across organizational boundaries and software applications, which can lead to expensive mistakes.

A healthcare enterprise has different facilities and systems that are used for processing patient data. A patient may receive care at more than one physical facility affiliated with the same organization, sometimes by random occurrence and sometimes as part of the medical management process. In such an instance, and when no data are exchanged between the facilities' systems or incomplete data exchange occurs between disjoint systems, the same patient may end up with two different identifiers or medical record numbers within one healthcare information system (HIS). The issue of dealing with duplicate data has pestered data warehouse initiatives for quite a while. Such situations require data cleansing, record cleanup, and record linkage efforts.

Chapter-3

Information Systems in Healthcare

❖ **Role of information systems in Modern Healthcare Environments**

The healthcare industry is always eager to put new digital solutions into practice to manage the financial, administrative, and clinical operations of healthcare institutions. Technology implementations have greatly benefited the fields of healthcare informatics, healthcare data, information technology, and business. Health information systems, or HIS for short, are a technological blessing for the healthcare sector that make managing patient data extremely effective.

⇨ Some of the key components of information systems in healthcare:

• **Core Administration Management**

In healthcare organizations, independent or cloud-based computer systems for health information technology frameworks serve as the primary administrative system. This system aids in recording and incorporating each department's daily operations within a healthcare system.

• **Financial Software Component**

Chief Financial Officers (CFOs), or those in charge of monitoring and controlling revenue cycles, use HIS software to carry out their management procedures and develop their strategies. SaaS accounting plug-ins and financial management are frequently connected to create a strong base for financial management services.

Ensuring that healthcare revenue cycles are properly monitored can improve resources and open up the ecosystem to spending more on software and operation tools that add value.

- **ERP/Personnel Management Tools**

Employee and patient management tools together assist the personnel management capabilities incorporated by Health Information System. These healthcare IT systems help in facilitating transparent resource allocation, communication, and scheduling of appointments between patients and providers across various facilities and departments. The major ERP system supplier strategically considers the healthcare potential of its growing market.

- **Documenting Medical Information**

EHR and EMR information systems help in tracking appointments of patients, financial information, care notes, etc., for dedicated documenting frameworks for implementing overall HIS in healthcare. This assists in ensuring high-priority documents from patient information to financial details are maintained across encrypted and secure health information system portals via proper accessibility control.

- **Tracking of Assets**

Healthcare administrative inventory management and monitoring are facilitated by medical inventory management systems, or asset tracking, from the point of purchase through the compensation process. With access tracking, an item in the inventory that is about to expire can be restocked and replenished while ensuring that best practices for inventory maintenance are adhered to.

- **Managing Medial Transportation**

Federal law in the United States mandates that health care information systems pay for the least expensive means of transportation for patients to and from medical appointments. This is especially valid for emergency medical transportation as well as non-emergency transportation. In order to support the HIS in the healthcare component, it must also keep up with the tracking, distribution, and upkeep of these vehicles.

Benefits of Health Information System

The benefits of health information technology is designed to store, manipulate, collect, and analyze patient information to support their decision-making process in healthcare facilities. In the present time, it has become a growing recognition as a potential benefit of HIS in healthcare.

- **Organized & Coordinated Treatment Process**

A technology-driven system called a health information system makes it simple for organizations and providers to share protected health information (PHI). Additionally, patients can receive seamless and well-coordinated treatment from healthcare providers thanks to this system. HIS is most beneficial to patients whose diagnoses require significant medical information management and cross-specialty treatment coordination. Above all, it enhances patient outcomes and the way that care is delivered.

- **Improved Patient Safety**

With the aid of health information systems, you can easily access patient data, save it all, and share it across several databases to increase patient safety. You will also receive alert notifications in the event that a patient's health is compromised. For instance, if a patient has a medication they are not prescribed, program security checking can notify healthcare providers of any potential negative effects the patient may have. By doing this, you can steer clear of any major errors that may arise from making decisions based on incomplete information.

- **Betterment in Patient Care**

By collecting and saving patients' information, including diagnosis reports, medical history, allergy reactions, vaccinations, treatment information plans, test results, etc., Health Information Systems provide healthcare providers with a complete and orderly framework that helps them interact with their patients in a better way and eventually deliver care to them in a more efficient way.

- **Hassle-free Process of Performance Analysis**

Using Health Information Systems enables multiple avenues through which you can access your staff performance, analyze patient care, and check the efficiency and stability of your organization. HIS reduces the paperwork and makes every record computerized. You can take any decision related to your staff based on their skill sets. Also, you can take decisions after focusing on previous performance details. With HIS, your patients get the chance of sharing reviews regarding the level of care they are receiving from your staff so that you can stay aware of the performance of your staff and analyze the effectiveness of your organization.

- **Transfiguration in Clinical Procedures**

With HIS, you can address any kind of stressful situation for your patients. You can have a virtual view of patient flow and what every individual patient experiences during their meeting with health care providers, administrative personnel, lab technician, and financial assistants. Careful attention to this helps you spot the areas where you can bring betterment.

- **Circumvention of Medical Errors**

As Health Information Systems maintain less paperwork and makes everything computerized and automated, you get error-free reports and information. As a result, various medication errors can be avoided and patients' safety can be ensured.

- **Instant & Seamless Accessibility to Patients' Details**

"The Health Information System collects data from the health sector and other relevant sectors, analyses the data and ensures their overall quality, relevance, and timeliness, and converts data into information for health-related decision-making," per a World Health Organization (WHO) report. Furthermore, you will have a better chance of making decisions, carrying out regulations, policies, and training and development initiatives, as well as conducting health research and monitoring service delivery, if the information is more trustworthy.

- **Minimized Operational Expense**

Health Information Systems Enable health organizations to assign resources in a planned manner and save potentially remarkable amounts of expenses, energy, and supplies. In a nutshell, you can make your healthcare service better for your patients while saving lots of money.

- **Saving of Time**

Health information systems not only save costs but also save time. HIS saves a great deal of time in coordinating patient care and streamlining hospital administration by digitizing all patient data and automating personal tasks.

- **Improved Patient Satisfaction**

Health Information Systems enhance the clinical process and increase patient satisfaction in addition to simplifying the daily tasks of healthcare administrators and providers. Patients can rely on your service, and as you establish yourself as a trustworthy brand in your industry, you attract more business and see excellent returns on your investment.

Important Features of Health Information Systems

- **Patient Portal**

One crucial component of the health information system is the patient portal. It is a platform that is comparable to an electronic health record, but it differs in that patients can use it to securely access their medical records online, make appointments, consult with doctors, check their bills, and make payments. To take full advantage of the feature, all they need is a smart device. Rather than going through the traditional process of making an appointment with their doctor, they can simply log in to the patient portal, check which of their doctors are available, and schedule an appointment that works for both of them. They can review the bill, make the payment, or establish the information for upcoming payments after setting up the appointment. Because it makes patients' treatment processes more transparent and increases their accessibility, the patient portal is becoming more and more popular every day. Hospitals choose to do this in order to increase patient satisfaction and establish their reputation as trustworthy facilities.

- **Medical Billing**

With the help of the online medical billing feature, all billing tasks are completed faster than before. The days of hospitals needlessly devoting a significant amount of time to scheduling and billing are long gone. Everything can now be managed effectively thanks to the medical billing feature, including patient billing, insurance information, patient tracking, and the payment procedure. In order for you to respond appropriately in the event of a payment delay or other problems, you can even receive a notification alert.

Moreover, the claim scrubbing tool in medical billing helps you detect any type of medical errors way before they start to slow down your management process. It includes scanning and getting rid of any LCD, CCI, or HIPAA-based errors, and delivering you the latest updated reports.

- **Patient Scheduling**

Similar to the patient portal, patients can book their own appointments through patient scheduling by just signing into their individual accounts. In this manner, they avoid having to stand in line outside the clinic or doctor's office or to keep calling the office to schedule an appointment. With just a tap, all the amenities will be accessible around-the-clock. They can even schedule appointments based on how convenient it is for them and the doctor's availability. The caregivers can also benefit from this feature. If necessary, they can assign their personnel, test facilities, and specialized equipment.

- **ePrescribing**

This software in Health Information Systems speeds up the complete prescription process, usually done by the staff members of the medical practitioner's office. They can send and fill the prescriptions of every patient to the pharmacies online. Also, they can track the entire process and take any action if needed. This way the whole process becomes quick, safe, and error-free.

- **Remote Patient Monitoring**

This is yet another exciting aspect of health information systems— it makes patient data easily accessible, aids in the provision of quality care by healthcare providers, and reduces costs associated with severe conditions. For patients with long-term medical conditions, remote patient monitoring, or RPM, is quite helpful. RPM data is gathered and used by doctors to track patients' health conditions. Additionally, with the help of these details, they are able to predict or prevent situations that otherwise would require urgent medical attention. RPM is useful in situations other than chronic health care, like caring for elderly patients, providing care following a patient's discharge, treating mental health and drug addiction issues, etc.

- **Master Patient Index**

Many hospitals and sizable organizations of medical practices use the Master Patient Index. The patient's information only needs to be input once using this technology. Subsequently, it is linked to various databases, which means that this information may prove helpful for additional laboratory tests and clinical divisions down the road. The data won't need to be manually entered each time. The primary advantage of utilizing the Master Patient Index is the convenience with which patient information can be accessed. It is also fully automated, which lowers the chance of mistakes and increases information security.

Chapter-4

Shared Care & Electronic Health Record

The use of shared electronic health records creates a wealth of new opportunities for adaptable and productive collaboration between medical staff members in various healthcare facilities, all to the benefit of the patients. Nonetheless, there are still unresolved security and legal issues.

Key challenges include:

(1) allocation of responsibility

(2) documentation routines

(3) and integrated or federated access control.

Shared Health Records (SHR)

Medical data can be shared between multiple health information systems thanks to shared health records, or SHR. By supporting better patient care, the exchange of this data leads to better health outcomes. Health data stored in an integrated data repository can be shared amongst different institutions and services through the use of shared health records. The standardized patient data is stored in the data repository; it is gathered from various sources, such as an Electronic Medical Record (EMR) or a Laboratory Information Management System (LMS). Medical facilities with the necessary authorization can update patient records. Users of a shared health record will have access to useful, real-time data.

The integration of shared electronic health records has given rise to a vast range of new opportunities in healthcare. It can foster productive collaboration among various health personnel in many health institutions. This type of progress will no doubt be of great help to patients. Unfortunately, there remains some unresolved security and legal concerns to be ironed out.

=> Benefits of a Shared Health Record

- It Stores Vital Data

Important information such as test results, care summaries, medical or nursing care plans, and allergies are kept in shared health records. For instance, an ultrasound picture with the patient's demographic data attached can be stored in shared health records. This is referred to as document-based data stored with its associated metadata in the medical field.

- Better Healthcare

Patients are able to receive better care because their healthcare staff will have quick and easy access to their records. This will help to improve many areas pertaining to patient care, such as patient-centeredness, timeliness, efficiency, communication, safety, effectiveness, education, and equity.

- Easy Retrieval of Data

A shared health record system facilitates easy retrieval of the necessary shared clinical record as needed. The users may also retrieve more than one document for one or more patients at the same time.

- Easy Data Update

Existing medical records within a shared health record system can easily be updated. Once new information (such as a blood test result) for a client is available, it can be entered into the system immediately.

- Reducing Costs of Resources

The use of shared health records has financial benefits for medical facilities and can continue to do so. They no longer have to print or copy paperwork to send to various medical facilities or departments. As a result, they can save money by having less paperwork. Additionally, patients can save money because sharing medical records can occasionally help to avoid repeat testing.

- Helpful for Research

The clinical data being stored can be used in studies and researches. Once the permission is given, then the researchers quickly and efficiently are provided with data to support their cause.

- Effective Written Communication

The healthcare team can document in a clear, accurate, and comprehensive manner thanks to the use of shared health records. The purpose of the shared health records system was to store copies of the data subsets that were collected by point of service (POS) applications. Data that are clinically relevant must be its main focus. The following is a list of the different kinds of information that can be stored in a shared health record system:

- Problems/Conditions/Diagnosis
- Care Plans
- Basic Encounter Information
- Referral Orders and Referral Notes
- Care Protocols
- Health Status indicators
- Encounter Summaries
- Clinical Observations

Challenges of Capturing Rich Patient Histories in a Computable Form

Information gathered during patient appointments is captured and managed using electronic health records, or EHRs. Personal health records (PHRs), patient portals, claims data, and payer reimbursement information are additional sources of data used to create patient profiles. Another initiative that speeds up the transfer and consolidation of data between different care partners is the health information exchange (HIE). In addition, a plethora of additional factors could influence health outcomes.

As one might imagine, bringing so much data together and using it to make decisions is not without challenges. Fragmented data, ever-changing data, privacy/security regulations and patient expectations are four of the primary data challenges facing the health care industry today.

1. Fragmented Data

A dizzying array of sources and formats, including structured data, paper, digital, images, videos, multimedia, and more, are used to collect health care data. The communities that collect and aggregate data are likewise dispersed, which makes it extremely difficult to extract and integrate data. Data is collected by payers, providers, employers, social networks, public health experts, and patients; however, there is no attempt to harmonize the data. There is no single source of truth; instead, there is data duplication and divergence.

This results in inaccurate and incomplete health care member profiles with little insight into a patient's well-being journey and a member's ever-evolving relationship with providers, payers, pharmacy, friends and family members. A lack of understanding, monitoring and support cause low adherence and high readmission risks. Poor communication (particularly during the preoperative phase) often results in cancellation of procedures, causing loss of revenue and inefficient resource utilization.

2. Ever-changing Data

Like everyone else, doctors and patients move, change their names and occupations, retire, and pass away. Payer organizations might also move, open new locations, or engage in different types of mergers and acquisitions. Furthermore, it can be difficult to maintain accurate, full, and up-to-date health care data due to changes in service delivery, medication delivery, and personalized care models. Providers' ability to remain in business and members' experiences are both directly impacted by outdated data and information latency. As a result, the implementation of new treatment options is delayed, health care programs are not adequately responded to, and patient engagement and experience are subpar.

3. Privacy and Security Regulations

Upholding patient trust is essential to creating a productive healthcare environment. Since patient privacy depends on HIPAA2 compliance and the safe adoption of electronic health records, data security has become crucial for the healthcare sector. Additionally, maintaining data sets and engagement compliant can be difficult due to constantly shifting regulatory requirements. Organizations are unable to comply with new regulatory requirements due to poor data quality and strategy, which also drives up the expense of audits and reporting. It will be difficult to improve public health until data security and compliance issues are sufficiently resolved.

4. Patient Expectations

The health care industry is about to experience the same shift we saw in retail, banking and hospitality. The health care system is on the verge of a perfect storm. A silver tsunami — in the form of the aging baby boomer population – will put the system through a stress test, while pressures from millennials and Generation Z will force health care organizations to choose newer forms of engagement. Health care organizations must equip themselves for a new age, volume and type of members. The industry will need to have an understanding of members' changing needs and their preferences and then provide solutions that align with their way of life.

Latest Global Developments and Standards to Enable Lifelong Electronic Health Records to be Integrated from Disparate Systems

The health care sector and the prospects for electronic health records have seen a lot of upheaval recently. The introduction of COVID-19 in recent years has demonstrated the importance of digital solutions in addressing the myriad problems that healthcare organizations face.

Virtual health adoption has become essential, particularly in light of COVID-19 restrictions that have compelled patients and healthcare providers to find innovative solutions. Virtual care is here to stay. Since their creation in the 1960s, electronic health records, or EHRs, have come a long way, but there is still much more that needs to be done.Here are some electronic health records trends to keep an eye out for in the coming years.

Integration and Interoperability

The inability of EMRs to integrate with other systems is a drawback. For example, in order to obtain a complete picture of a patient's health, a hospital needs records from outpatient practices and any other hospitals the patient has visited in the past. EMRs have not historically been interoperable. Consequently, an EHR system should be chosen over an EMR system by any organization seeking this feature.

EHRs are expected to be updated to comply with interoperability policies in the upcoming year, as they offer more robust capabilities and can integrate with patient portals.

As the demand for interoperability grows, the line between EMRs and EHRs continues to blur. Many use the terms interchangeably even though, historically, interoperability was a major distinguisher between the two. So while vendors may refer to a product as an EMR, they're increasingly becoming closer to what were originally EHRs.

Although there are some interoperability problems in cloud infrastructures too, they are widely used in the health care industry today. A cloud EHR that offers a pay-as-you-go option for providers helps them operate with limited budgets. This can enable people with less spending capacity to afford EHRs in lieu of buying EMRs in case they have interoperability as a must-have feature on their list.

Furthermore, the cloud environment allows providers to offload the security responsibility to some extent. The majority of cloud EHR providers offer expert security programs and round-the-clock support to guarantee the security of protected health information (PHI) at all times.

Blockchain technology can be applied to improve semantic interoperability. Blockchain does away with the requirement for expensive EHR integrations. To access a patient's documents, a private key is the only requirement. Without the need for integrations, a medical professional with legitimate credentials might be able to access health records at any time and from any place.

Cloud Computing

Staff shortages are one of the top challenges medical facilities have faced since the start of the COVID-19 pandemic. This is giving rise to cloud computing as medical organizations can start drifting towards outsourcing administrative and clinical services, including medical billing, reporting, lab integration and more.

Standardization

The Office of the National Coordinator for Health Information Technology oversees the standardization of EHR regulations. Practices risk fines and loss of meaningful use eligibility if their EHRs don't meet those requirements.

The main factor driving their growth is the development and standardization of APIs, which allow for rapid information exchange and access between various parties.

The guideline mandates that all electronic health information (EHI) pertaining to a patient, regardless of its structure, must be freely accessible via electronic means.

Robotic Process Automation

The global market for automated data capture for electronic medical records is growing as a result of improved workflows and increased accuracy. Robot-based automation, or robotic process automation (RPA), circumvents the need for human entry, helping to achieve the necessary accuracy.

RPA is a method used in healthcare to address EHR shortcomings without completely rebuilding the system's architecture. RPA primarily makes it possible to use digital labor to keep things working while fixing deeper issues.

RPAs use system algorithms and programs to safely and effectively automate the processes that an organization's human resources would typically carry out through manual efforts. These help medical facilities accelerate digitization and imperfections in absolutely no time.

Telehealth

Clinical workflows are enhanced and remote care is made possible for medical organizations by integrating EHR systems with telehealth platforms. Physicians can quickly and securely transfer patient data between systems (or interfaces) thanks to these integrations. EMR systems and telehealth collaborate incredibly well to deliver excellent patient care in a remote setting. Some of the greatest advantages that you and your employees can obtain together are listed below:

- Automate data entries
- Synchronize insurance information in a single window
- Streamline virtual care activities
- Enhance patient-physician engagement
- Boost collaboration

Modifying information in the telehealth system automatically updates patient records to give providers immediate access to up-to-date and accurate patient information during virtual care.

IoT, AI & Voice Recognition

Several practices also integrate artificial intelligence to help physicians diagnose and identify patient health trends. Many companies are researching to add voice recognition using AI to EHR software.

In addition, integrating natural language processing (NLP) into EHR systems will improve physician efficiency and patient treatment. AI systems that use natural spoken language to understand physicians are the future.

Artificial intelligence technology is being used in the healthcare industry to improve the efficiency of electronic systems. This allows medical professionals and caregivers to swiftly review and evaluate unstructured patient cases using automation tools. This also makes it easier for administrative staff to quickly preauthorize insurance without running into problems or inconsistencies in the process.

Healthcare workers can benefit from artificial intelligence in many ways. In addition to creating customized lesson plans to offer comprehensive support with therapies and treatments, it looks through patient databases to give doctors timely feedback while handling urgent patient cases involving uncommon or complicated medical conditions.

Error Reduction

With paper prescriptions, patients blamed physicians for illegible handwriting errors. Computer-based charts have reduced mistakes, but reliance on digitalization can cause problems with dependency on computers to supply correct dosages.

Physicians receive too many notifications from EHR systems, which makes them less attentive to patients. This is one problem that needs to be addressed. Practitioners are overwhelmed by the volume of message alerts and patients' demands for immediate communication. This can result in errors and issues because sending messages and sifting through several notifications can cause one to predictably forget important things. Errors have detrimental effects and can lower the standard of care and medication provided to patients.

Blockchain and EHR

Although blockchain technology is more well-known for its part in cryptocurrencies, it has recently found application in the medical field. Blockchain secures EHR data with cryptography, making it accessible only to authorized users.

Blockchain, for instance, can monitor medication distribution, verify prescription authenticity, validate clinical trial and claim results, and stop insurance fraud. Blockchain can also be used by smart contracts to reduce human intervention by acting on predefined outcomes. Although the use of blockchain technology is still in its infancy, a number of EHRs have integrated it to guarantee security, scalability, and confidentiality.

5G, 6G and Big Data

Everyday interactions on the Internet of Things (IoT) exchange huge amounts of data. The availability of 5G data has provided a phenomenal increase in internet speeds and device loads impacting all facets of data, software and how people interact with devices. Due to its high data output, 5G can positively influence automation tools, enabling them to produce faster than they do today.

The next big thing coming soon is 6G, which will increase transmission bandwidth.Given that it is currently in the development stage and is scheduled for delivery by December 2023, we should be able to witness its rapid advancements altering the landscape of EHR/EMR systems by 2024.

Big data analytics has the potential to significantly improve the health care sector. It will significantly aid in the improvement of telehealth services, resulting in better analysis reports and patient treatment procedures with reduced diagnostic costs. Advanced data mining techniques and analysis tools available in big data can also help treat rare diseases.

Wearable Devices

Overall, the amount of connected wearable devices is expected to surge in the coming years. Data integration from wearable devices to EHR systems offers opportunities to provide better patient care. Wearable devices, more popularly known as wearables, have sensors that measure activity levels, steps walked and other environmental indicators. They come in many forms, including smart-watches, smart goggles and fitness trackers, and push the data to apps on users' mobile phones.

These tech devices offer users detailed insights into several months of information, including day-to-day activities, health conditions, medication routines and more. With technological advancements, these gadgets now let health care facilities, including caregivers and doctors, remotely monitor the health of their high-risk patients around the clock.

Real-time Data and Analytics

Medical facilities amass enormous volumes of patient information. Clinical decision support (CDS) is a service that vendors provide to physicians based on patient health and financial data. Issues with accessibility related to interoperability can be resolved by utilizing analytics algorithm predictions. Data warehouse development offers the chance to guarantee cleaner patient data because of automation.

Chapter-5

Patient Safety & Clinical Risk

Patient Safety

The growing complexity of healthcare systems and the consequent increase in patient injury in healthcare facilities gave rise to the medical specialty of patient safety. Its goal is to stop and lessen the risks, mistakes, and harm that happen to patients while receiving medical care. Continuous improvement based on learning from mistakes and unfavorable events is a cornerstone of the field.

In order to provide essential health services of high quality, patient safety is paramount. In fact, there is broad agreement that effective, secure, and person-centered healthcare should be provided everywhere. In addition, timely, equitable, integrated, and efficient health services are necessary to achieve the advantages of high-quality healthcare.

To ensure successful implementation of patient safety strategies; clear policies, leadership capacity, data to drive safety improvements, skilled health care professionals and effective involvement of patients in their care, are all needed.

Clinical Risk

Clinical risk includes any undesirable situation or operational factor that may have negative consequences for patient safety or capable of causing an adverse event (AE). The AE, intentional or unintentionally, may be related to the human factor, that is, medical errors (MEs).

⇨ **Relationship between Patient Safety & Informatics**

The 21st century has seen a tremendous shift in healthcare due to technological advancements. Although the use of electronic health records (EHRs) has a major influence on this, other technologies have also surfaced that are improving patient safety and health outcomes while also increasing the efficiency of healthcare.

Wearable medical technology, interoperable systems, and telehealth and telemedicine are some of these innovations. Strong ties between medical professionals and health IT specialists are necessary to effectively implement this new technology and guarantee that patient safety and medical staff are supported.

The impact of health information technology on patient safety and care is as varied as the systems and devices now in use. However, much of it starts with the adoption of EHR by medical facilities in the last decade. These records provide a central repository of a patient's medical history, allowing for the sharing of clinical information, including physician notes, test results, and information on prescription drugs.

EHR's take into account the impact of human factors in healthcare, improving communication and providing "one source of truth" on patient health and treatment for better coordination of the patient care process.

Information technology's influence now extends beyond data visibility and sharing to include using data for patient care that is informed by data. Improving patient safety increasingly depends on advanced data analytics. With analytics programs able to generate COVID-19 patient risk profiles that more accurately identified those most at risk of fatal outcomes in the early stages of the pandemic, the coronavirus pandemic has highlighted the significance of health data. Because there is such a wide range of technology available, health IT specialists and leaders in the healthcare industry must use an organized method to apply the technology that best suits their particular needs. The Institute for Healthcare Improvement states that comprehending these three important aspects of healthcare technology will help you make the most out of this.

1. Understanding Needs

Administrators, clinical leaders and IT leaders must come together to identify areas where technology will benefit their specific operation, then set goals for what they want to achieve with that technology.

2. Asking the Right Questions

Both health IT professionals and clinicians must consider every potential tech solution through the lens of how it will impact the work of clinicians, lead to improved patient care and safety, and ultimately, positive health outcomes.

3. Bringing Health IT and Health Clinicians Together

Asking the right questions is dependent on health clinicians and health IT coming together for greater coordination between the work each group does. That's the best way to get on the same page about how to approach integrating technology. For example, having IT personnel attend clinical meetings could provide greater insight into medical operations.

Information Technology with the Greatest Impact on Patient Safety

Easier Access to Information

Health IT specialists have spent years working on interoperability, or the capacity to share patient data across various systems. As these digital systems advance, physicians will be able to share patient data, reducing the possibility of treating a patient incorrectly. For example, a hospital doctor has access to a patient's personal physician's records. It can also be useful in warning medical professionals at the earliest stages of a pandemic, as the COVID-19 emergency has shown.

Adoption of Digital Medical Records

The work responsibilities of nurses and other staff members have been significantly impacted by electronic medical and health records. It is now required of nurses to know how to enter patient data into the system. Medical coders maintain the appropriate codes current in the records. These documents are also used by the billing department to file insurance claims. In general, patients receive better, more effective care when their medical records are digital.

Reduction of Drug-Related Errors

Mistakes in prescribing drugs is a medical error with potentially catastrophic consequences. Electronic prescribing has helped to mitigate risks in this area. These systems reduce the potential for medication errors by moving handwritten scripts to electronic entry on a secure device, automatically checking for drug interactions, automating re-fill requests and reminders, as well as raising alerts if a suspected error is made in the prescribing or administering of medication.

Improved Public Health

Public health involves creating preventive programs that help people stay healthy longer, as well as identifying chronic health issues within specific population demographics. In focusing on the overall population, public health informatics utilizes data from a variety of sources—including hospitals, social services, surveys and more—to help healthcare providers and government agencies address and prepare for new health threats.

For example, data in EHR is extremely valuable in applying

analytics in population health management, allowing researchers to detect a problem early (such as flu outbreak) and act quicker (in the case of flu, getting more vaccines into the affected community).

Clinical Decision Support

One of the most important areas where technology can increase patient safety is in clinical decision support (CDS). With CDS, a clinician can access all pertinent patient data in real-time, along with codified standards regarding possible treatments, thanks to technology.

The Agency for Healthcare Research and Quality (AHRQ) reports that there were "increased clinical practice guideline use and concordance, improved care process measures, and reduced safety events" in a review of CDS in oncology care.

The Future of Information Technology and Patient Safety

⇨ Artificial intelligence (AI) and machine learning have far reaching potential and still un-tapped applications in many industries, and healthcare is no exception.

⇨ In that same report from AHRQ, it noted that AI can enhance and expand CDS. For example, AI systems currently under development can detect complex conditions such as sepsis or other warning signs of patient deterioration, according to the report.

⇨ AI and machine learning also can play a role in the business of healthcare. Advanced systems can handle many of the routine processes in billing and coding, freeing up humans to take on more complex jobs.

⇨ Another area to emerge in recent years is predictive health analytics. Advanced systems will eventually be able to prescribe the best course of a treatment for a patient and compare potential outcomes based on different options available for clinicians.

⇨ Advances in technology will continue to drive the future of healthcare. For those with a desire to be on the frontlines in applying technology towards improving patient safety and health outcomes, graduate certificate and degree programs in health informatics and healthcare analytics can provide the knowledge needed to lead in the field.

Nursing Informatics & Patient Safety

The rapidly evolving field of nursing informatics is revolutionizing the way nurses provide patient care. Healthcare informatics, clinical informatics, patient safety, health information management, and other fields are all included in the broad field of informatics, which is the application of computing technology to healthcare. This article will go over how monitoring vital signs and assisting in the identification of possible safety hazards can help to improve patient safety. When defining nursing informatics, the American Nurses Association's (ANA) definition is frequently cited:

Nursing Informatics "is the specialty that integrates nursing science with multiple information and analytical sciences to identify, define, manage, and communicate data, information, knowledge, and wisdom in nursing practice."

Nursing informatics professionals are, first and foremost, patient advocates. Patient safety is their number one priority, and they work with a diverse group of stakeholders across the care continuum to bridge the gap between clinical and technical perspectives. This field has helped drive healthcare's application of technologies such as Electronic Medical Records (EMRs) and computerized provider order entry.

They are in charge of creating and putting into place sophisticated nursing information systems and technology, as well as policies and procedures that support initiatives for quality improvement, evidence-based practice, care coordination, and the best possible results.

By giving nurses the resources they need to recognize and control risks, nursing informaticists can contribute to increased patient safety. For instance, if a patient's vital signs are not stable, this can be a sign that a major health issue is about to arise. Tools funded by nursing informatics can be used by nurses to track their progress toward patient safety objectives, make patient safety plans, and keep an eye on vital signs.

Some mobile system helps hospitals improve patient safety across the enterprise with minimum impact on the alarm burden and clinical workflow. If we can help nurses detect patient deterioration early enough, further complications can be avoided. It is designed to provide continuous surveillance monitoring for patients in general care settings and beyond.

With continuous surveillance monitoring of key vital signs, early recognition and detection of patient deterioration enable clinicians to make timely and effective interventions.

Mobile monitors the following:

- Arrhythmias
- Posture
- Skin Temperature
- Continuous Non-Invasive Blood Pressure
- Heart Rate
- Pulse Rate
- SpO2
- Posture
- Respiration Rate

- Fall Detection

Functions & Applications of Risk Management Process

The methods and procedures used in healthcare facilities to identify, reduce, and eliminate risks are collectively referred to as healthcare risk management. Recognize its goals, components, the responsibility of the risk manager, and more.

The clinical and administrative systems, procedures, and reports used in healthcare risk management are used to identify, track, evaluate, reduce, and eliminate risks. Healthcare organizations protect patient safety and their assets, market share, accreditation, reimbursement levels, brand value, and reputation by proactively and methodically implementing risk management.

Deployment of healthcare risk management has traditionally focused on the important role of patient safety and the reduction of medical errors that jeopardize an organization's ability to achieve its mission and protect against financial liability. But with the expanding role of healthcare technologies, increased cyber security concerns, the fast pace of medical science, and the industry's ever-changing regulatory, legal, political, and reimbursement climate, healthcare risk management has become more complex over time.

⇨ To navigate the healthcare risk continuum healthcare organizations and risk managers need to:

•**Identify Risk** It is difficult to identify every threat a healthcare organization faces because risk management entails managing uncertainty and new risk is always emerging. However, by utilizing data, institutional and industry knowledge, and involving all relevant parties (payers, employees, administrators, and patients), healthcare risk managers are able to identify potential compensatory events and threats that would otherwise be difficult to predict.

• **Quantify & Prioritize Risk** Once identified, it is vital to score, rank, and prioritize risks based on their likelihood and impact of occurrence and then allocate resources and assign tasks based on these measures. To accomplish this, risk matrices and heat maps can be deployed that will also help to visualize risks and promote communication and collaborative decision-making.

• **Investigate & Report Sentinel Events** Coined by the Joint Commission, Sentinel Events are "any unanticipated event in a healthcare setting resulting in death or serious physical or psychological injury to a patient or patients, not related to the natural course of the patient's illness." When a sentinel event occurs, quick response and thorough investigation address immediate patient safety issues and reduce future risk. Having an established plan in place promotes calm and measured response and transparency by staff and ensures that corrective actions can be implemented and evaluated. Sentinel events are not always the result of errors. However, achieving transparency and thorough evaluation requires healthcare organizations to establish an atmosphere of respect, trust, and cooperation between staff and leadership.

• **Perform Compliance Reporting** As with the Joint Commission, Federal, state, and other oversight bodies mandate reporting of certain types of incidents including sentinel events, medication errors, and medical device malfunctions. Incidents such as wrong-site or patient surgery, workplace injuries, medication errors, etc. need to be documented, coded, and reported.

• **Capture & Learn from *Near Misses & Good Catches*** When mistakes or adverse events are avoided due to luck or intervention, "near misses" and "good catches" occur. These are often the best way to identify and prevent risk. Healthcare providers should develop a culture that encourages reporting so that prevention measures and best practices can be instituted.

• **Think Beyond the Obvious to Uncover Latent Failures** When a nurse administers the incorrect dosage of medication to a patient, for instance, it is clear and simple to spot an active failure. Conversely, latent failures are frequently concealed and can only be found by careful investigation and analysis. Was it difficult to read the patient's chart due to dim lighting? Did the nurse rush because he had too many patients with high levels of acuity? Examine both underlying and less obvious causes when investigating an unpleasant episode.

•**Deploy Proven Analysis Models for Incident Investigation** To comprehend latent failures and causes as well as relationships among risks, accident analysis models are utilized. For instance, medical errors are frequently caused by understaffing and fatigue. The efficacy and efficiency of risk management are increased by using proven models. The Sharp and Blunt End Assessment of Clinical Errors model and the are two accident analysis models used in healthcare risk management. Both Root Cause Analysis and FMEA, or Failure Mode and Effects Analysis, are used in conjunction with comprehensive frameworks to help identify the causes and consequences of medical errors.

• **Invest in a Robust Risk Management Information System (RMIS)** Multiple platforms for reporting and managing risk are on the market. These systems provide tools for documenting incidents, tracking risk, reporting trends, benchmarking data points, and making industry comparisons. Reports can be generated for losses, incidents, open claims, and lost work time for injured employees to name a few. RMIS can greatly enhance risk management by improving performance through available and reliable systems while providing overall cost reduction by automating routine tasks.

• **Find the Right Balance of Risk Financing/ Transfer/ Retention** Risk financing involves an organization's methods for efficiently and effectively funding loss that results from risk. It includes risk transfer usually through insurance policies and risk retention such as self-insurance and captive insurance.

⇨ The format of a Risk Management Plan varies by organization and is contingent on the analysis of existing systems and historical data as well as the unique characteristics of each healthcare entity. That said, there are some fundamental components that belong in all healthcare risk management plans:

• **Education & Training** The requirements for employee training, which should include orientation for new hires, continuous and in-service training, an annual competency review and validation, and training specific to events, must be outlined in risk management plans.

• **Patient & Family Grievances** Procedures for recording and handling patient and family complaints should be outlined in the risk management plan in order to improve patient satisfaction and lower the possibility of legal action. It is necessary to clearly define and convey response times, staff duties, and recommended actions.

• **Purpose, Goals, & Metrics** Risk management plans should clearly define the purpose and benefits of the healthcare risk management plan. Specific goals to reduce liability claims, sentinel events, near misses, and the overall cost of the organization's risk should also be well-articulated. Additionally, reporting on quantifiable and actionable data should be detailed and mandated by the plan.

• **Communication Plan** The healthcare risk management plan should include information about how and with whom to communicate about risk, even though the team's promotion of candid and spontaneous dialogue is crucial. Documentation of next actions and follow-up tasks is necessary. The plan must also specify the reporting obligations to departments and C-Suite executives. In addition, anonymous reporting features and a safe, "no-blame" culture should be encouraged by the plan.

• **Contingency Plans** Risk management plans also need to include contingency preparation for adverse system-wide failures and catastrophic situations such as malfunctioning EHR systems, security breaches, and cyber attacks. The plan needs to include emergency preparedness for things like disease outbreaks, long-term power loss, and terror attacks or mass shootings.

• **Reporting Protocols** Every healthcare organization must have a quick and easy-to-use, system for documenting, classifying, and tracking possible risks and adverse events. These systems must include protocols for mandatory reporting.

• **Response & Mitigation** Plans for managing healthcare risk must also incorporate cooperative mechanisms for handling risks and incidents that are reported, such as acute response, follow-up, reporting, and preventing repeat failures.

Chapter-6

Clinical Knowledge & Decision Making

Role of Knowledge Management

For over fifty years, critical thinking has been emphasized in nursing education as a critical nursing skill. Over time, definitions of critical thinking have changed. There are a few important definitions of critical thinking to take into account. Critical thinking is described as deliberate, self-regulatory judgment that makes use of cognitive tools like interpretation, analysis, evaluation, inference, and explanation of the evidentiary, conceptual, methodological, criteriological, or contextual considerations that form the basis of the judgment (American Philosophical Association, APA).2. In summary, self-directed, self-disciplined, self-monitored, and self-corrective thinking can be summed up as a more comprehensive general definition of critical thinking.

It presupposes assent to rigorous standards of excellence and mindful command of their use. It entails effective communication and problem solving abilities and a commitment to overcome our native egocentrism and sociocentrism. Every clinician must develop rigorous habits of critical thinking, but they cannot escape completely the situatedness and structures of the clinical traditions and practices in which they must make decisions and act quickly in specific clinical situations.

There are three key definitions for nursing, which differ slightly. Bittner and Tobin defined critical thinking as being "influenced by knowledge and experience, using strategies such as reflective thinking as a part of learning to identify the issues and opportunities, and holistically synthesize the information in nursing practice". Scheffer and Rubenfelexpanded on the APA definition for nurses through a consensus process, resulting in the following definition:

In order to provide high-quality nursing care and maintain professional accountability, critical thinking is crucial for nurses. These mental habits are displayed by critical thinkers in the nursing profession: self-assurance, perspective on the larger picture, inventiveness, adaptability, curiosity, intellectual honesty, intuition, open-mindedness, persistence, and introspection. The cognitive abilities of analysis, standard application, discrimination, information seeking, logical reasoning, prediction, and knowledge transformation are practiced by critical thinkers in the nursing field.

The National League for Nursing Accreditation Commission (NLNAC) defined critical thinking as:

The deliberate nonlinear process of collecting, interpreting, analyzing, drawing conclusions about, presenting, and evaluating information that is both factually and belief based. This is demonstrated in nursing by clinical judgment, which includes ethical, diagnostic, and therapeutic dimensions and research.

These concepts are furthered by the American Association of Colleges of Nurses' definition of critical thinking in their Essentials of Baccalaureate Nursing:

Critical thinking underlies independent and interdependent decision making. Critical thinking includes questioning, analysis, synthesis, interpretation, inference, inductive and deductive reasoning, intuition, application, and creativity.

Course work or ethical experiences should provide the graduate with the knowledge and skills to:

- Use nursing and other appropriate theories and models, and an appropriate ethical framework;
- Apply research-based knowledge from nursing and the sciences as the basis for practice;
- Use clinical judgment and decision-making skills;
- Engage in self-reflective and collegial dialogue about professional practice;
- Evaluate nursing care outcomes through the acquisition of data and the questioning of inconsistencies, allowing for the revision of actions and goals;
- Engage in creative problem solving

When considered collectively, these critical thinking definitions outline the range and essential components of the mental processes involved in delivering clinical care. The definition of critical thinking will have an impact on how it is taught and what level of care nurses are expected to provide.

The inclusion of critical thinking in all nursing curricula has been mandated by professional and regulatory bodies; however, the distinction between critical reflection and ethical, clinical, or even creative thinking for decision-making or actions that the clinician is required to take has not been sufficiently made. Under the umbrella of critical thinking, other crucial ways of thinking, like clinical reasoning, evidence evaluation, creative thinking, or the application of accepted standards of practice, have been included. These are all separate from critical reflection. Critical thinking and clinical reasoning and judgment are frequently confused in the literature on nursing education.

The accrediting bodies and nursing scholars have included decisionmaking and action-oriented, practical, ethical, and clinical reasoning in the rubric of critical reflection and thinking. One might say that this harmless semantic confusion is corrected by actual practices, except that students need to understand the distinctions between critical reflection and clinical reasoning, and they need to learn to discern when each is better suited, just as students need to also engage in applying standards, evidence-based practices, and creative thinking.

Higher-order thinking abilities are required due to the expanding body of research, patient acuity, and complexity of care. Using information and experience to pinpoint patient issues and guide clinical decisions and actions that lead to better patient outcomes is known as critical thinking. Teachers who exhibit the qualities of critical thinking—independence of thought, intellectual curiosity, courage, humility, empathy, integrity, perseverance, and fair-mindedness—can foster these abilities in their students.

The process of critical thinking is stimulated by integrating the essential knowledge, experiences, and clinical reasoning that support professional practice. The emerging paradigm for clinical thinking and cognition is that it is social and dialogical rather than monological and individual.Clinicians pool their wisdom and multiple perspectives, yet some clinical knowledge can be demonstrated only in the situation (e.g., how to suction an extremely fragile patient whose oxygen saturations sink too low). Early warnings of problematic situations are made possible by clinicians comparing their observations to that of other providers. Clinicians form practice communities that create styles of practice, including ways of doing things, communication styles and mechanisms, and shared expectations about performance and expertise of team members.

Students can easily misunderstand the logic and goals of various modes of thinking if they use critical thinking as a broad umbrella for them. Multiple thinking skills, including critical thinking, clinical judgment, diagnostic reasoning, deliberative rationality, scientific reasoning, dialogue, argumentation, creative thinking, and so forth, are essential for both scientists and clinicians. Clinicians in particular need to be proactive and to continuously grasp the trajectory of a patient's health status and care needs. This calls for critical reflection, critical reasoning, clinical judgment, and an assessment of their own clarity and understanding of the current situation.

Critical Reflection, Critical Reasoning, and Judgment

Examining the underlying presumptions and seriously challenging the veracity of claims, arguments, and even case facts are necessary components of critical reflection. Although critical reflective skills are vital for clinicians, they are insufficient for the clinician who has to make decisions about how to act in specific situations to prevent harm to patients. In everyday practice, for instance, when attempting to determine the deviations from the typical, well-grounded understanding that has existed since Harvey's work in 1628, clinicians cannot afford to critically reflect on the well-established tenets of "normal" or "typical" human circulatory systems.

Yet critical reflection can generate new scientifically based ideas. For example, there is a lack of adequate research on the differences between women's and men's circulatory systems and the typical pathophysiology related to heart attacks. Available research is based upon multiple, taken-for-granted starting points about the general nature of the circulatory system. As such, critical reflection may not provide what is needed for a clinician to act in a situation. This idea can be considered reasonable since critical reflective thinking is not sufficient for good clinical reasoning and judgment. The clinician's development of skillful critical reflection depends upon being taught what to pay attention to, and thus gaining a sense of salience that informs the powers of perceptual grasp. The powers of noticing or perceptual grasp depend upon noticing what is salient and the capacity to respond to the situation.

While critical reflection is an important professional skill, clinicians also need to be able to reason and use logic. The capacity for critical thought informs decision-making through inference, deduction, analysis, questioning presumptions, and assessment of available data and information.Critical reasoning is the process of applying knowledge and experience to weigh several options for achieving the desired outcomes while taking the patient's circumstances into account. Both deductive and inductive cognitive abilities are employed in this process. Clinical reasoning is occasionally described as a means of assessing scientific information or even as a type of scientific reasoning. Making good clinical decisions requires critical thinking.

An essential point of tension and confusion exists in practice traditions such as nursing and medicine when clinical reasoning and critical reflection become entangled, because the clinician must have some established bases that are not questioned when engaging in clinical decisions and actions, such as standing orders. The clinician must act in the particular situation and time with the best clinical and scientific knowledge available. The clinician cannot afford to indulge in either ritualistic unexamined knowledge or diagnostic or therapeutic nihilism caused by radical doubt, as in critical reflection, because they must find an intelligent and effective way to think and act in particular clinical situations. Critical reflection skills are essential to assist practitioners to rethink outmoded or even wrongheaded approaches to health care, health promotion, and prevention of illness and complications, especially when new evidence is available. Breakdowns in practice, high failure rates in particular therapies, new diseases, new scientific discoveries, and societal changes call for critical reflection about past assumptions and no-longer-tenable beliefs.

Unlike other forms of reasoning, clinical reasoning is situated and practice-based. It is more dependent on prior knowledge about general cases from scientific and technological research than it is on any one specific instance. Understanding the evidence supporting general scientific and technical knowledge and how it relates to a specific patient also requires practical ability. While making these decisions or drawing conclusions, the clinician takes into account the patient's unique clinical trajectory, their concerns and preferences, as well as their unique vulnerabilities (such as having multiple comorbidities) and sensitivities to care interventions (such as known drug allergies, other conflicting comorbid conditions, incompatible therapies, and past responses to therapies).

Situated in a practice setting, clinical reasoning occurs within social relationships or situations involving patient, family, community, and a team of health care providers. The expert clinician situates themselves within a nexus of relationships, with concerns that are bounded by the situation. Expert clinical reasoning is socially engaged with the relationships and concerns of those who are affected by the caregiving situation, and when certain circumstances are present, the adverse event. Halpern has called excellent clinical ethical reasoning "emotional reasoning" in that the clinicians have emotional access to the patient/family concerns and their understanding of the particular care needs. Expert clinicians also seek an optimal perceptual grasp, one based on understanding and as undistorted as possible, based on an attuned emotional engagement and expert clinical knowledge.

The wisdom of expanding their limited understanding of rationality beyond straightforward rational calculation (as demonstrated by cost-benefit analysis) has begun to be recognized by clergy educators, nursing educators, and medical educators. They have come to reconsider the necessity of character development, which includes emotional engagement, perception, thought habits, and skill acquisition, as crucial to the development of expert clinical reasoning, judgment, and action. Like the clergy, practitioners in the fields of engineering, law, medicine, and nursing must establish a position for themselves within their discipline's scientific and knowledge-based traditions in order to identify and assess important evidence at the time it is needed. Both disciplinary nihilism and diagnostic confusion pose a threat to a clinician's ability to act in specific circumstances.

However, the practice and practitioners will not be self-improving and vital if they cannot engage in critical reflection on what is not of value, what is outmoded, and what does not work.

Clinical judgment requires clinical reasoning across time about the particular, and because of the relevance of this immediate historical unfolding, clinical reasoning can be very different from the scientific reasoning used to formulate, conduct, and assess clinical experiments. While scientific reasoning is also socially embedded in a nexus of social relationships and concerns, the goal of detached, critical objectivity used to conduct scientific experiments minimizes the interactive influence of the research on the experiment once it has begun. Scientific research in the natural and clinical sciences typically uses formal criteria to develop "yes" and "no" judgments at prespecified times. The scientist is always situated in past and immediate scientific history, preferring to evaluate static and predetermined points in time (e.g., snapshot reasoning), in contrast to a clinician who must always reason about transitions over time.

Techne and Phronesis

Aristotle first examined the differences between techne and phronesis, or the mere scientific making of things, and practice. Developing the moral imagination necessary for good practice is a necessary part of learning to be a good practitioner. Practitioners must use moral imagination to determine the likely reason behind a patient's treatment refusal, for instance, if the patient exercises their right to refuse. Was the rejection, for instance, motivated by delusions, irrational fears, misinterpretation, or even clinical depression?

Techne, as defined by Aristotle, encompasses the notion of formation of character and habitus as embodied beings. In Aristotle's terms, techne refers to the making of things or producing outcomes. Joseph Dunne defines techne as "the activity of producing outcomes," and it "is governed by a means-ends rationality where the *maker or producer* governs the thing or outcomes produced or made through gaining mastery over the means of producing the outcomes, to the point of being able to separate means and ends". While some aspects of medical and nursing practice fall into the category of techne, much of nursing and medical practice falls outside means-ends rationality and must be governed by concern for doing good or what is best for the patient in particular circumstances, where being in a relationship and discerning particular human concerns at stake guide action.

Phronesis, in contrast to techne, includes reasoning about the particular, across time, through changes or transitions in the patient's and/or the clinician's understanding. As noted by Dunne, phronesis is "characterized at least as much by a perceptiveness with regard to concrete particulars as by a knowledge of universal principles". This type of practical reasoning often takes the form of puzzle solving or the evaluation of immediate past "hot" history of the patient's situation. Such a particular clinical situation is necessarily particular, even though many commonalities and similarities with other disease syndromes can be recognized through signs and symptoms and laboratory tests. Pointing to knowledge embedded in a practice makes no claim for infallibility or "correctness." Individual practitioners can be mistaken in their judgments because practices such as medicine and nursing are inherently underdetermined.

Phrenetic knowledge cannot continuously surpass the institutional setting's capabilities and supports for best practices, even though it must be open to revision and improvement, actual occurrences, and consequences. Phronesis also depends on the practitioner's continued experiential learning, in which information is improved, updated, or disproved. Practical knowledge and experiential learning were devalued in the Western tradition, which valued knowledge that could be applied to all situations, with the notable exception of Aristotle. This preference for formal logic and reasoned calculation was formalized by Descartes.

Aristotle recognized that when knowledge is underdetermined, changeable, and particular, it cannot be turned into the universal or standardized. It must be perceived, discerned, and judged, all of which require experiential learning. In nursing and medicine, perceptual acuity in physical assessment and clinical judgment (i.e., reasoning across time about changes in the particular patient or the clinician's understanding of the patient's condition) fall into the Greek Aristotelian category of phronesis. Dewey sought to rescue knowledge gained by practical activity in the world. He identified three flaws in the understanding of experience in Greek philosophy:

(1) empirical knowing is the opposite of experience with science;

(2) practice is reduced to techne or the application of rational thought or technique;

(3) action and skilled know-how are considered temporary and capricious as compared to reason, which the Greeks considered as ultimate reality.

Both techne and phronesis are necessary in the practice of nursing and medicine. As demonstrated by standardized blood pressure readings, diagnoses, and even patient condition and treatment charts, the clinician routineizes and standardizes what can be routineized and standardized. Except for the necessary timing and modifications made for specific patients, procedural and scientific knowledge can frequently be formalized and standardized (e.g., practice guidelines) or at least made explicit and certain in practice.

Rational calculations available to techne—population trends and statistics, algorithms—are created as decision support structures and can improve accuracy when used as a stance of inquiry in making clinical judgments about particular patients. Aggregated evidence from clinical trials and ongoing working knowledge of pathophysiology, biochemistry, and genomics are essential. In addition, the skills of phronesis (clinical judgment that reasons across time, taking into account the transitions of the particular patient/family/community and transitions in the clinician's understanding of the clinical situation) will be required for nursing, medicine, or any helping profession.

Thinking Critically

Critical thinking skills allow nurses to meet patients' needs in the context of their choices, in the face of uncertainty, and by considering other options. This leads to the provision of higher-quality care and allows nurses to think critically as opposed to accepting orders and carrying out tasks without careful thought or analysis. The cognitive abilities of skilled practitioners include information searching, discriminating, analyzing, transforming knowledge, predicating, applying standards, and logical reasoning. These abilities enable them to think critically. Age, length of education (e.g., associate vs. baccalaureate decree in nursing), and completion of philosophy or logic subjects can all have an impact on an individual's capacity for critical thought.

The skillful practitioner can think critically because of having the following characteristics: motivation, perseverance, fair-mindedness, and deliberate and careful attention to thinking.

Thinking critically implies that one has a knowledge base from which to reason and the ability to analyze and evaluate evidence. Knowledge can be manifest by the logic and rational implications of decisionmaking. Clinical decisionmaking is particularly influenced by interpersonal relationships with colleagues, patient conditions, availability of resources, knowledge, and experience. Of these, experience has been shown to enhance nurses' abilities to make quick decisions and fewer decision errors, support the identification of salient cues, and foster the recognition and action on patterns of information.

In order to recognize and comprehend the needs and concerns of their patients, clinicians must cultivate the interpersonal and character traits necessary for this. Accurate interpretation of patient data that is pertinent to the particular patient and circumstance is necessary for this. In the context of nursing, developing moral agency involves learning to be accountable in the specific ways that the profession requires, as well as being able to observe and discern changes in patients' concerns and/or clinical conditions that call for action from nurses or other healthcare professionals in order to prevent possible compromises to the quality of care.

Formation of the clinician's character, skills, and habits are developed in schools and particular practice communities within a larger practice tradition. As Dunne notes,

A practice is not just a surface on which one can display instant virtuosity. It grounds one in a tradition that has been formed through an elaborate development and that exists at any juncture only in the dispositions (slowly and perhaps painfully acquired) of its recognized practitioners. The question may of course be asked whether there are *any* such practices in the contemporary world, whether the wholesale encroachment of Technique has not obliterated them—and whether this is not the whole point of MacIntyre's recipe of withdrawal, as well as of the post-modern story of dispossession.

Clearly Dunne is engaging in critical reflection about the conditions for developing character, skills, and habits for skillful and ethical comportment of practitioners, as well as to act as moral agents for patients so that they and their families receive safe, effective, and compassionate care.

While professional socialization and values are important, they fall short in addressing the development of character and skills that change how a practitioner lives in the world, what the practitioner can observe and react to based on ingrained emotional response patterns, skills, acting dispositions, and the ability to respond, decide, and act. What distinguishes a practice from being just a technical, repetitive manufacturing process is the requirement for the clinician to develop their character and skills.

In nursing and medicine, many have questioned whether current health care institutions are designed to promote or hinder enlightened, compassionate practice, or whether they have deteriorated into commercial institutional models that focus primarily on efficiency and profit. MacIntyre points out the links between the ongoing development and improvement of practice traditions and the institutions that house them:

The corrupting of traditions is a result of a lack of justice, truthfulness, courage, and the necessary intellectual virtues. It also affects institutions and practices that draw their existence from the traditions they represent in the modern era. Naturally, acknowledging this also means acknowledging the existence of another virtue—the virtue of having a sufficient understanding of the traditions one is a part of or must contend with—whose significance is perhaps most evident when it is least evident. This virtue is not to be confused with any form of conservative antiquarianism; I am not praising those who choose the conventional conservative role of laudatory temporize act. It is rather the case that an adequate sense of tradition manifests itself in a grasp of those future possibilities which the past has made available to the present. Living traditions, just because they continue a not-yet-completed narrative, confront a future whose determinate and determinable character, so far as it possesses any, derives from the past.

Without real-world practice scenarios and specific patient cases, it would be impossible to capture all the situated and distributed knowledge. Because simulations allow students to practice in a more simplified setting, they are effective teaching tools for fostering critical thinking skills in nurses. However, when a lot of the information is based on perceptions of various patient aspects and changes that have occurred over time, students may find it difficult to convey underdetermined situations. The subcultures that emerge in practice environments and establish the social climate of competence, mistrust, trust, scarce resources, and other types of situated possibilities are not possible to recreate in simulations.

Experience

A qualitative study of adult, pediatric, and neonatal intensive care unit (ICU) nurses, where the nurses were clustered into advanced beginner, intermediate, and expert level of practice categories, is one of the hallmark studies in nursing that offers keen insight into understanding the influence of experience. With up to six months of work experience, the advanced beginner used protocols and procedures to decide which clinical actions were necessary. The advanced beginner believed their practice was unsafe due to a lack of knowledge or a confusion in applying knowledge when faced with a complex patient situation. When they gained experience in real-world clinical settings and had access to knowledge from their peers' mistakes, they started to evolve from advanced beginners to competent practitioners.

Competent nurses continuously questioned what they saw and heard, feeling an obligation to know more about clinical situations. In doing do, they moved from only using care plans and following the physicians' orders to analyzing and interpreting patient situations. Beyond that, the proficient nurse acknowledged the changing relevance of clinical situations requiring action beyond what was planned or anticipated. The proficient nurse learned to acknowledge the changing needs of patient care and situation, and could organize interventions "by the situation as it unfolds rather than by preset goals. Both competent and proficient nurses (that is, intermediate level of practice) had at least two years of ICU experience. Finally, the expert nurse had a more fully developed grasp of a clinical situation, a sense of confidence in what is known about the situation, and could differentiate the precise clinical problem in little time.

Expertise is a mark of a nurse who has progressed beyond proficiency and is obtained through professional experience. Experience, according to Gadamer, entails refuting prior beliefs and understandings while also deepening or expanding upon knowledge. According to Dewey, an enhanced environment and a ready "creature" are necessary for the experience. Experiential learning can be explained, expanded upon, or even refuted by the chance to reflect on and tell the story of what one has learned.

Experiential learning requires time and nurturing, but time alone does not ensure experiential learning. Aristotle linked experiential learning to the development of character and moral sensitivities of a person learning a practice. New nurses/new graduates have limited work experience and must experience continuing learning until they have reached an acceptable level of performance.After that, further improvements are not predictable, and years of experience are an inadequate predictor of expertise.

Over time, the most proficient creator and scholar of applied knowledge establishes a continuous conversation and link between the lessons learned during the day and hands-on learning. In a late-life interview, Gadamer emphasized the ongoing and flexible character of experiential learning with the following response:

Being experienced does not mean that one now knows something once and for all and becomes rigid in this knowledge; rather, one becomes more open to new experiences. A person who is experienced is undogmatic. Experience has the effect of freeing one to be open to new experience.

In our experience we bring nothing to a close; we are constantly learning new things from our experience this I call the interminability of all experience.

Practical endeavor, supported by scientific knowledge, requires experiential learning, the development of skilled know-how, and perceptual acuity in order to make the scientific knowledge relevant to the situation. Clinical perceptual and skilled know-how helps the practitioner discern when particular scientific findings might be relevant.

Experimentation confirms experience and knowledge, which are frequently viewed as opposites and presented as either-or options. In actuality, though, it is widely accepted that scientific inquiry and subsequent experiential learning are both fueled by experiential knowledge. Learning firsthand from specific clinical cases can inspire new scientific inquiries and research as well as assist the clinician in identifying similar cases in the future. Nursing diagnoses practice guidelines, for instance, can be used by less experienced nurses—and, one could argue, experienced nurses as well—to further their careers. Their assessment of the needs, reactions, and circumstances of the patients is reflected in the guidelines, which necessitates critical thought and judgment.Following rules also shows that one can recognize problems and solve them.On the other hand, the hallmark of expertise is the capacity to carry out a number of tasks competently without the need for nursing diagnoses.

Experience precedes expertise. As expertise develops from experience and gaining knowledge and transitions to the proficiency stage, the nurses' thinking moves from steps and procedures (i.e., task-oriented care) toward "chunks" or patterns(i.e., patient-specific care). In doing so, the nurse thinks reflectively, rather than merely accepting statements and performing procedures without significant understanding and evaluation. Expert nurses do not rely on rules and logical thought processes in problem-solving and decision making Instead, they use abstract principles, can see the situation as a complex whole, perceive situations comprehensively, and can be fully involved in the situation. Expert nurses can perform high-level care without conscious awareness of the knowledge they are using and they are able to provide that care with flexibility and speed. Through a combination of knowledge and skills gained from a range of theoretical and experiential sources, expert nurses also provide holistic care.Thus, the best care comes from the combination of theoretical, tacit, and experiential knowledge.

It is believed that experts eventually acquire the capacity to instantly identify crucial elements of the circumstance and to know instinctively what to do.There have been suggestions that expert nurses offer patients high-quality care, but this has not always been proven, especially when it comes to patient outcomes. Additionally, the differences in the effects of care provided by "expert" nurses are not well understood. In fact, a number of studies have shown that performance metrics and outcomes are frequently unrelated, or even negatively related, to the duration of professional experience.

In a review of the literature on expertise in nursing, Ericsson and colleagues found that focusing on challenging, less-frequent situations would reveal individual performance differences on tasks that require speed and flexibility, such as that experienced during a code or an adverse event. Superior performance was associated with extensive training and immediate feedback about outcomes, which can be obtained through continual training, simulation, and processes such as root-cause analysis following an adverse event. Therefore, efforts to improve performance benefited from continual monitoring, planning, and retrospective evaluation. Even then, the nurse's ability to perform as an expert is dependent upon their ability to use intuition or insights gained through interactions with patients.

Intuition and Perception

The instantaneous comprehension of information devoid of rational thought processes is known as intuition. In clinical practice, intuition, according to Young, is the process by which a nurse perceives something about a patient that is hard to express. Factual knowledge, "immediate possession of knowledge, and knowledge independent of the linear reasoning process" are attributes of intuition. When intuition is employed, information that was first sparked by the imagination is filtered, allowing for the integration of all available knowledge and data to solve problems.

Clinicians use their interactions with patients and intuition, drawing on tacit or experiential knowledge, to apply the correct knowledge to make the correct decisions to address patient needs. Yet there is a "conflated belief in the nurses' ability to know what is best for the patient" because the nurses' and patients' identification of the patients' needs can vary.

King and Appleton conducted a review of the literature and rhetoric on intuition and discovered that all nurses, including students, used intuition (i.e., gut feelings). They discovered evidence that intuition was activated in response to knowledge and that it served as a catalyst for action and/or reflection that directly affected the analytical process involved in patient care. This evidence was primarily found in critical care units. The difficulty faced by nurses stemmed from the fact that strict adherence to guidelines, checklists, and standardized documentation overlooked the advantages of intuition. Rew and Barrow supported this viewpoint in their reviews of the literature, finding that intuition was unrelated to physiological measures, difficult to measure and assess quantitatively, and essential to complex decisionmaking.

Intuition is a way of explaining professional expertise. Expert nurses rely on their intuitive judgment that has been developed over time.Intuition is an informal, nonanalytically based, unstructured, deliberate calculation that facilitates problem solving, a process of arriving at salient conclusions based on relatively small amounts of knowledge and/or information. Experts can have rapid insight into a situation by using intuition to recognize patterns and similarities, achieve commonsense understanding, and sense the salient information combined with deliberative rationality. Intuitive recognition of similarities and commonalities between patients are often the first diagnostic clue or early warning, which must then be followed up with critical evaluation of evidence among the competing conditions. This situation calls for intuitive judgment that can distinguish "expert human judgment from the decisions" made by a novice.

Role of Knowledge Management in Improving Decision Making

Every one of the 67 million or so people who call the United Kingdom home will work in the health industry at some point in their lives. The healthcare industry depends heavily on knowledge for day-to-day operations. In particular, the provision of quality patient outcomes depends on the cooperation of multiple partners who exchange knowledge.

Treating an individual patient is dependent on accessing a huge amount of knowledge and expertise, and healthcare providers must not only share clinical knowledge but also standard operating procedures. Information is constantly changing as the medical field evolves, with new research published and as new treatments become available.

Need of healthcare knowledge management

"Doctors and medical personnel are overloaded," is the succinct reply. The paradox is that despite being overloaded with information, healthcare professionals find it difficult to find. Compare this to the reality that timely access to the right information can literally save lives.Assume you work as a doctor and see dozens of patients every day. Physicians make decisions based on their own experience as well as the scant patient data at their disposal.

There's no time in a patient's appointment to track down another doctor, who are probably all busy with their own patients. In a scenario where a patient comes to their doctor with symptoms that are perplexing, the doctor makes an educated guess as to what may be wrong and writes a treatment plan for the patient.

To help the patient, it would be much more beneficial if the physician had access to the knowledge of all other medical professionals in the hospital in addition to their own expertise. It's possible that another physician has seen a patient with a bewildering set of symptoms before and can offer guidance on what to do next.

This is where healthcare knowledge management comes in. Doctors can use it to search for symptoms and other valuable data that will make a huge difference to outcomes for their patients.

Many businesses are already using knowledge management systems to organize, store, and share knowledge between employees and boost operational efficiency. These systems are increasingly being used by healthcare organizations to raise the standard of care for patients.

In the medical field, having access to the appropriate information is crucial because a patient's life may be at risk. Systems for managing knowledge facilitate practitioner collaboration and increase knowledge availability across the entire organization.

Importance of knowledge management in healthcare

Information is currency in the healthcare industry. It's an intangible asset that helps strengthen and develop a strong organization even though its market value may not reflect it. Employees who are overly knowledgeable, however, may become overwhelmed and unsure of where to begin their search for solutions.

It's crucial to organize this knowledge in such a way as to make it manageable for your practitioners. The knowledge that is not accessible is of no use to anyone.

KM can be seen under two dimensions- internal knowledge management for healthcare workers to understand protocols, new studies, and research, documentation on processes, and procedures. Another one is to help serve patients with better knowledge of customers, knowledge about customers, and knowledge from customers.

Benefits of knowledge management in healthcare

The use of knowledge management in healthcare has many benefits. We'll go through some of them now.

Avoid malpractices

Medical malpractice can be prevented when knowledge is accurately recorded and practitioners are aware of the need to adhere to established protocols. Following step-by-step procedures helps practitioners to provide better care by lowering the possibility of error. There are consequently fewer incorrect diagnoses because they have access to the expertise of other practitioners.

Informed decision making

When employees have better access to information they can make more informed decisions when it comes to patient care. Practitioners aren't just making decisions based on their own experience, but they can learn from the knowledge of others. They know they have access to the most up-to-date knowledge that has been recorded by their fellow practitioners based on their extensive experience in the healthcare field.

Educate and empower medical practitioners

Sharing knowledge helps medical professionals become more knowledgeable and capable by allowing them to benefit from the practice's collective experience. Employees provide better care and patient outcomes are enhanced when they are given the freedom to learn from the most recent information available in the field. Diagnoses made by patients shift from conjecture to reliance on the most recent information provided by their peers.

Capture tactical knowledge gained by practitioners

When knowledge management software is used properly it can capture practical knowledge gained by practitioners and promote a culture of continuous learning. The expertise can be made available to everyone in the practice who can apply that learning to their own dealings with patients.

Boost operational efficiency

By providing knowledge to everyone, you can prevent your staff from constantly having to start from scratch. Any question that arises has undoubtedly already been addressed by someone within the company, and knowledge management systems can aid in the documentation of answers. By leveraging the prior experiences of others, practitioners can increase operational efficiency.

Improve patient satisfaction

Patients experience better results and are happier with the care they received when your practitioners are more productive. Knowledge management is all about keeping the patient at the center of everything that occurs within the company and improving service delivery as a result.

Leads to digital transformation

Electronic medical recordkeeping has already replaced paper recordkeeping in healthcare organizations. The introduction of digital systems results in better patient care as well as increased productivity and efficiency, but the change doesn't end there.

A healthcare knowledge base is a crucial part of healthcare organisations meeting their digital innovation goals and it doesn't have to be a painful process. Healthcare workers can collaborate more efficiently, leading to enhanced patient outcomes. The solution should offer robust search, and integrate with other apps, in order to fit into the provider's existing workflows.

Promotes collaboration between healthcare workers

Instead of using paper files that are easily lost or damaged, patient medical records are now stored almost universally in an electronic format. It's easy for doctors to search for files, make updates, and share records. It's much more efficient, and protects patient/doctor confidentiality.

A knowledge base is a secure way to share information about patients while honouring patients' privacy. Medical professionals can collaborate on sharing symptoms, treatments, and other information while keeping individual patient records confidential.

Implementing a new knowledge base

1. Evaluate your needs and pain points

Before starting the process of adopting a new knowledge base, a plan must be created. Similar to how one wouldn't embark on a trip without a plan, healthcare institutions should identify the major issues and opportunities that are necessitating the adoption of new technologies. Determine the meaning of "value" within your company. A new digital solution should ideally reduce expenses for the team and benefit users in a way that justifies the initial investment in technology.

2. Assemble a team of diverse stakeholders and experiences

Everyone is going to be impacted by new technologies. A cross-functional group can convene and resolve concepts prior to submitting the project proposal to upper management. With mergers and acquisitions still having an impact on the healthcare industry, a diverse stakeholder team can guarantee that digital transformation initiatives are implemented consistently throughout recently merged systems.

3. Balance your objectives for success

When choosing your new knowledge base, you should evaluate your objectives. These objectives should be people, process, and technology. You must identify individuals who are responsible for delivering and receiving services, address security and usability, and adopt new tools to improve service delivery for patients and staff. This three-pronged approach can work for projects of any size.

4. Prepare yourself for roadblocks

Change takes time and there will inevitably be problems in the way. Transitioning from legacy systems is not easy and people are often resistant to change. Don't forget to focus on the small wins and their role in bringing about the larger end goal.

Features of knowledge management tools in healthcare

We'll now go over some common features of KMSs that you may find useful in the medical field. A search bar in your knowledge management tool will help practitioners quickly locate information in the knowledge base. It should predict what users will type as they input a search term and return the search results in a matter of seconds. The results should be sorted by relevance and contain keywords from both the title and the body of the article.

Interactive knowledge base

Users should be able to interact with your knowledge base, which should include engaging videos and images. To help practitioners feel like your knowledge management system is the center of a community, allow users to post comments and take part in discussions about the content.

Challenges that limit KM implementation in healthcare

Lack of leadership

The leadership team should support the delivery of knowledge management in the healthcare industry. Initiatives related to knowledge management will not take off without the support of management and will not be embraced by all members of your workforce. Senior management should be the ones to lead by example when it comes to sharing knowledge and inspire the rest of the team to do the same.

Organizational culture

Sometimes you may run into friction at a culture level, which means it takes a long time to implement any KM initiatives. You may lack resources needed to launch knowledge management, and employees may have conflicting goals which make it hard to get started with KM.

Lack of organizational structure

Knowledge management relies on having a strong organizational structure that enables employees to find their role in the dissemination and consumption of knowledge. Without proper structure in place, employees are confused about the roles they should play and knowledge management initiatives will fail.

Limited tech infrastructure

In certain healthcare organizations, implementing digital knowledge management systems can be challenging due to limited technological infrastructure. Knowledge management is a technology-intensive field that necessitates individual workers' skills in order to initiate projects. Teams with even the most basic infrastructure can use knowledge management tools if they select the right ones, which can be available as a subscription-based service that just requires an internet connection.

Lack of methodology

Your knowledge management efforts will come to a standstill if you don't have a well-defined process for gathering and organizing knowledge. To manage your knowledge systems, you must have a well-thought-out plan and appoint the appropriate personnel. It is important to adhere to the proper protocols in order to promote knowledge sharing.

Lack of knowledge management strategy

Knowledge management needs to be backed by a solid strategy, and without one initiatives are left being directionless and aimless. The strategy needs to take into account people, processes and tools in order to be successful. You should have someone leading the strategy and organizing others who need to be involved.

The attitude of physicians and staff toward KM

If your doctors and other staff members have a hostile attitude, it could be difficult to implement knowledge management. Their culture might encourage knowledge hoarding rather than sharing, and they might not be inclined to share knowledge. Employees may not like being asked to work in new or different ways and may be resistant to the necessary changes.

Knowledge Management Best Practices for Healthcare

Virtual discussion forums

Encourage staff members to interact with one another in online discussion boards. They can exchange best practices for knowledge management as well as knowledge. Discussion boards will boost employee involvement and give them a greater sense of ownership over your knowledge management system.

Peer review and collaboration

For accuracy, every piece of content added to your knowledge base ought to undergo peer review. Content must be produced collaboratively because no one should be uploading to your system without first having their work reviewed. Features that enable a strict editing process and let you assign users to different roles should be included in your knowledge base.

Collect feedback

Knowledge management in healthcare is an ongoing process. In order to check you're going in the right direction, it's vital to collect feedback from practitioners on the quality and helpfulness of the content. Feedback can be as simple as asking your users to rate the helpfulness of the page they're on, to collecting qualitative feedback through forms, comments and surveys.

Knowledge map

A knowledge map is a visual representation of all the knowledge contained within your organization. It also helps identify those individuals who have relevant expertise and where they can be found. Using knowledge mapping is a vital tool in your knowledge management strategy.

Measure the metrics

Track performance using the metrics provided by your knowledge base software. Metrics can be used, for instance, to monitor author, article, and category performance. You can find out which articles are most popular with users, which require editing, and which are doing well. In addition to finding out which search terms yield no results, you can determine which authors are contributing the most popular articles, which can inspire you to create new content.

The Systematized Medical Nomenclature for Medicine–Clinical Terminology

A comprehensive, multi-hierarchical clinical terminology system is called Systematized Medical Nomenclature for Medicine–Clinical Terminology (SNOMED CT). It offers a consistent and empirically supported method for expressing clinical data. The potential applications of SNOMED CT are extensively documented, with multiple guides outlining different forms of implementation, including data aggregation, analysis, clinical records, and knowledge representation. In particular, the literature from earlier times outlines the different SNOMED CT development objectives. SNOMED CT, for instance, can be a standard used in electronic health records (EHRs) to code or classify clinical data. Standardized terminology also facilitates data storing, retrieval, and indexing.

This supports sharing of patient information across medical domains and organizations in ways that promote continuity of care. As a large-scale terminology system, SNOMED CT also enables knowledge representations in clinical guidelines and care pathways, which can be used, for example, with decision support.

Data recorded in EHRs are primarily used to provide care to patients. The potential of SNOMED CT to improve data quality and facilitate interoperability, and thus improve patient safety, has long been noted in existing research. Studies have shown that structured and standardized EHRs also increase data reuse possibilities. The European Union and the US Healthcare Information Technology Standards Panel have noted possibilities provided by SNOMED CT and taken steps toward increasing semantic interoperability, reuse, and the exchange of health data. Data recorded in local systems can also be used to support the achievement of broad health policy goals. The importance of SNOMED CT is expected to gradually grow, but at the same time, there is a need to tackle the complex implementation challenges that may arise.

SNOMED CT is used to consistently and fully represent clinical information when it is implemented in EHRs. SNOMED CT is used in more than 50 countries, but there aren't many published reviews about its clinical use, even though EHRs that are certified to adhere to terminology standards are widely used. The majority of research has been done on theory and predevelopment/design. Furthermore, research on the adoption of EHRs has previously examined broad factors, but it has not examined the variables linked to the implementation of less sophisticated EHR products in contrast to more sophisticated and established EHR systems. The maturity of an EHR system is relevant to appropriately maximize the benefit from prior experiences when implementing SNOMED CT.

In summary, even though SNOMED CT has been extensively studied as a clinical terminology system, previous research has repeatedly documented a lack of detailed evidence for SNOMED CT in clinical use cases. Considering that implementing SNOMED CT is a challenging proposition, the identification of specific barriers and facilitators to implementing SNOMED CT in clinical use is of paramount importance to further promote its adoption. Evidence from use cases might supportimplementation and provide guidance on avoiding deployment pitfalls. Therefore, we aimed to explore the available evidence in previous literature reviews of clinical use cases of SNOMED CT integrated into EHR systems or clinical applications during the last 5 years of continued development.In this study, we apply categories from previous research for analyzing use purpose and use phase for the terminology. Moreover, we present core benefits by summarizing the observations from the EHR use cases.

To explore EHR-related SNOMED CT use cases in recent research, our research team set out to conduct a systematic literature review. Our team consisted of a medical expert with decades of experience in clinical care and two health and medical informatics experts. To analyze EHR use cases where SNOMED CT terminology was applied, we extended the concept of EHR systems to cover EHR-related applications and software in clinical use. The word "clinical" refers to "medical work or teaching that relates to the examination and treatment of ill people". In our review, a use case consisted of SNOMED CT integrated into an EHR system in various stages of use, either in preuse development or in design, piloting, testing, implementation, use, or postimplementation evaluation.

The team followed the Cochrane review protocol to plan the necessary steps for this study design. Within the team, the application of the protocol was modified step-by-step to fit the research problem by first defining the search strategy, identifying the articles for the review by isolating the exclusion and inclusion criteria for assessing the search results, and lastly evaluating and summarizing the review results.

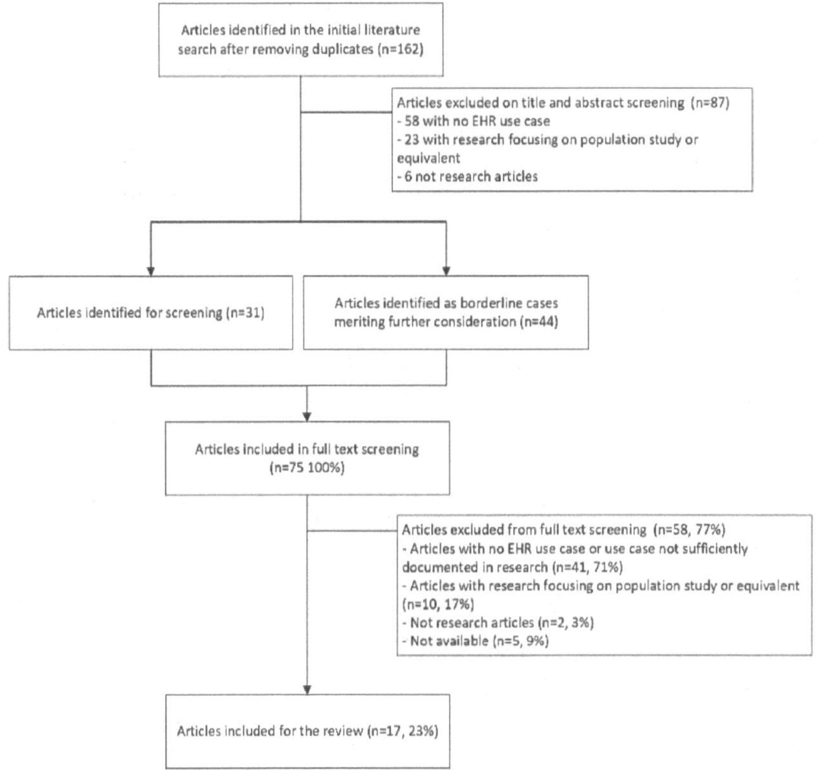

Fig- Application of the review protocol as a flowchart.

EHR: electronic health record.

By adding different search terms and comparing their appropriateness to the search results, we were able to define our search strategy. Numerous search results were returned when the keywords "EHR," "EMR," "electronic health record," or "electronic health record system" were entered. When these terms were combined with "SNOMED CT," pertinent search results were obtained for our review. Additionally, there was no discernible difference in the search results after adding filters. In March 2022, a systematic-review methods filter search was conducted on PubMed, yielding 162 original articles after duplicates were eliminated. Since our findings encompass the last five years of research, our review builds upon earlier reviews.

Prior to starting the search, the exclusion and inclusion criteria were established. Our criteria were developed based on prior research as well as our research questions. The following is how we defined the exclusion criteria: Initially, an EHR use case where SNOMED CT was being tested, piloted, implemented, or used in a clinical setting had to be documented in the original article. For instance, studies focusing on the theoretical development, assessment, or validation of SNOMED CT were not included in this. Second, we excluded population studies and, for example, cohort studies where SNOMED CT was used to define, extract, and harmonize study data and where no EHR-related design or use goals were documented. Third, we excluded editorials, posters, and other such sources to limit the review to original research articles. While reading the articles, we discussed how well the exclusion criteria corresponded to the delimitation made based on our research questions and the conclusions we arrived at while reading the research content as presented in the original articles.

We had eliminated 87 articles after the initial exclusion based on article headings and abstracts. Thirty-one articles that appeared to be relevant to our research question were included. Additionally, 44 cases that were on the borderline should be given extra thought to decide whether to include or exclude them. The goal for the two researchers was to read 75 full-text articles in all.

Contextual Factors of the Clinical Use Cases

The majority of the articles had inadequate descriptions of the EHRs, and there was no consistent framework for the detailed descriptions of the EHRs. As a result, the results are descriptive in nature. The precise product was only mentioned in one of the publications. The study focused on a high-maturity electronic health record (EHR) that supported care coordination and continuity of care, and was a comprehensive hospital information system. A prehospital patient record that wasn't connected into the hospital's electronic health record (EHR) was one of the systems. A primary care electronic health record (EHR) was one system that general practitioners used, and the other comprised integrated software for clinical use. Six systems were hospital EHRs. Among the system types were also the following: an "outpatient and inpatient EHR," a "centralized EHR with web-interface," and a "local EHR." One of the use cases described the system generally as an "ehr."

We examined the professional groups engaged in each use case to confirm the clinical orientation of the cases even more. The professional groups intended to use SNOMED CT (e.g., nursing informatics, medical informatics, or multi-professional users) were not explicitly stated, despite the fact that users were described. In seven of the use cases, the users were described in detail. Four cases were applied by physicians, by nurses, and 1 by physicians and nurses. Two of the cases were applied by a multi-professional team of clinicians, clinical and medical informatics professionals, clinical domain experts, terminologists, and clinical coders. Two of the articles specifically concerned clinical coders. Two of the remaining cases were generally described as having been applied by "clinicians." Four of the cases concerned researchers themselves, for whom specific clinical backgrounds were not reported.

SNOMED CT use purpose

Every piece of data explained one or more uses for the terms. Clinical needs for standardizing patient information were usually the driving force behind the adoption of SNOMED CT as standard terminology in the EHR. The main use purpose of the terminology as it is integrated or being implemented into an EHR is specifically referred to by the SNOMED CT use purpose in this instance. SNOMED CT, which is a common standard for EHRs, was the most frequently used category of use purpose. The objective of standardizing SNOMED CT in a different clinical application that is integrated with the EHR system was explained in two more studies. The use cases described communication and coordination needs, such as between hospital units or between inpatient and outpatient care, with the goal of promoting more reliable continuity of care and ultimately a higher quality of care. Accurate and timely diagnosis information with SNOMED CT deployment was reported as a crucial clinical need since it is major information in patient care. In 2 of the studies, SNOMED CT was implemented into the documentation of the problem list to increase the usefulness of the patient information and to organize the problem list content. Additionally, SNOMED CT was used to ensure effective data migration between systems.

According to different study materials, the main use purpose was to obtain or evaluate patient data for clinical research. This improved the sharing, retrieval, and analysis of data for clinical research among several hospitals. Common data models and terminology enabled distributed analysis and multisite data sharing. A medical annotation toolkit with a web interface for extracting necessary concepts was used in these two use cases. Two more studies concentrated on data extraction, classifying and coding patient data for research using SNOMED CT. The use purpose in these 2 studies was building clinical pathways and patient selection criteria based on terminology coding. Natural language processing of clinical, pathology, and genomics data was used for further clinical research. Moreover, the use cases illustrated the challenges of data sharing between inpatient care and a virtual hospital visit.

Two of the original articles focused on demonstrating the value of using SNOMED CT terminology in a clinical setting, and they described, to some extent, the already established use of the tool. Although there are many causes for inadequate clinical coding of patient data even after 20 years of EHR use, two primary ones are insufficient training and motivation. Domain-specific development, for instance, can advance support tools for the interoperable recording of patient information related to diagnosis, treatment, and interventions. One of the papers stated that the development of SNOMED CT was motivated by automated clinical coding. The development of computer-assisted coding may, through careful review and validation, improve the productivity of clinical coders. Different classificationsystems, such as the International Classification of Diseases–10, are typically linked and mapped to SNOMED CT for suitability in clinical use.

SNOMED CT Use Phase

The research team discussed these categories during the analysis because the phase of use was identified in the literature with varying degrees of accuracy. All 17 publications(100%) included clinical use phase documentation, albeit in vague ways. SNOMED CT in development was the most frequently used category of use phases, as evidenced by the six articles (6/17). It was anticipated that development would take several years because it was defined as an iterative process of analysis, validation, and standardization or creating and mapping EHR-structured content that needs cooperation and communication between stakeholders to improve the quality of care.

SNOMED CT in use was identified as the use phase in 5 EHR-related use cases and in implementation in 4 use cases . In the EHR-related use cases, SNOMED CT had been chosen as the base terminology system in the EHR or in a specific domain documented in the research to improve clinical information recording and coding, develop clinical pathways, and extract clinical data. The implementation cases addressed specifically improved the clinical recording of patient data by supporting clinicians' language and semantic selection with SNOMED CT or with a combination of SNOMED CT and other classification or terminology systems. Furthermore, two articles discussed the benefits of using SNOMED CT through post-implementation evaluation or a more proven merit approach, and one article described a pilot use of SNOMED CT in EHR use cases. The pilot case assessed instances where clinical data was either missing or incorrectly labeled due to, for instance, the use of abbreviations or nonstandard concepts. The purpose of the SNOMED CT use evaluation was to ascertain the effectiveness of fully integrated EHR services in patient care as well as the effects of recording clinical meanings with SNOMED CT. The secondary use purpose for using patient information was mentioned as an additional benefit.

Core Benefits of SNOMED CT

The research team compiled the main advantages of SNOMED CT, as shown in the 17 use cases, into a summary. The group classified the advantages using prior research as a guide. The main advantages had to do with the results of terminology use. With eight articles, improved data quality was the most frequently occurring category. The breadth and depth of the nomenclature served as the foundation for semantic-level fundamental benefits. SNOMED CT supported both the preferred language and the standardization of clinical meaning in the use cases. Custom concept dictionaries or language-specific subsets were constructed for a selected language for clinical use. Further benefits of implementing SNOMED CT were 2-fold: the parallel development of EHR technology and standardization. One UK use case documented evidence of increased interface usability and user satisfaction by clinicians. However, clinicians reported that adopting a new approach for data recording was a gradual process requiring time.

The benefits of providing a standardized method for indexing, storing, retrieving, and aggregating clinical data were covered in four articles. One use case focused on the advantages related to retrieving data. Benefits that have been documented indicated that more thorough clinical event documentation is needed. In order to support safe patient care, these benefits relied on the ability to access more comprehensive and coherent patient information, regardless of where it was recorded.

Summary of Findings

17 publications were found to have applied and utilized SNOMED CT in a clinical setting within EHRs or related clinical applications. Our goal was to ascertain whether enough research had progressed to permit a change in emphasis from reviews that have already been published and that discussed possible applications to studies that show real-world advantages of SNOMED CT. We present results from ongoing efforts over the last five years regarding the core benefits, use

phases, and clinical use purposes of SNOMED CT. These review categories have their roots in earlier studies that gave this analysis a solid foundation.

The use purpose for SNOMED terminology based on previous research was identified in all the articles reviewed. As we evaluated the use cases, these categories served our research material well. The most applied use purpose category was SNOMED CT as the planned standard for EHRs or other related applications. Other frequently applied use categories were the goals of using SNOMED for retrieving and analyzing patient data or implementing the terminology to advance the coding of patient data. Only 2 of the articles in the review entailed proof of merit of EHR implementation as the use purpose category. Based on these results, the initial observation was that there might be a level of interconnectedness between the use purpose and use phase. To prove this, data on the maturity of EHR solutions are needed to research the possible interconnectedness of EHR use and SNOMED CT. Moreover, it might be relevant to analyze relationships between use purpose and use phase. This requires testing the categories and their possible relationships with different data sets.

With respect to the use phase outcomes, every article that was reviewed provided an account of the SNOMED CT use phase; however, there were differences in the specifics of relevant contextual factors, like the clinical setting. This made it more difficult to evaluate the use phase's overall picture. Based on the findings, this could be a characteristic of this particular material, as it is typical of SNOMED CT use cases related to EHRs. Therefore, it could be beneficial in the future to focus especially on the descriptions of these kinds of SNOMED CT use cases. We suggest providing a more contextualized and structured description of the use phase. The scalability of the use-case results would increase with this level of accuracy. Lee et al have already highlighted that only a few SNOMED CT implementation cases are being published in the scientific literature. Through the systematic investigation of previous theoretical work , and with time, more comparable scientific publications on SNOMED CT use cases in a clinical context could be published.

Our review indicates that there is currently a dearth of research on the advantages of clinical SNOMED CT use in EHR-related use cases. We determined that the enhancement of data quality and the provision of a standardized method for indexing, storing, retrieving, and aggregating clinical data were the two most commonly mentioned categories of core benefits. Improvements in care quality with the aim of improving patient safety and, based on improved data quality, facilitating better continuity of care, were closely associated with these advantages. The review also discovered specific comments on enhancing coding productivity through automation or by providing clinical users with terminological support.

Such tools had potential to increase user satisfaction, although there was evidence for a need to involve clinicians from different domains in development. Evidence of practical advancement may motivate various clinical specialties to become more involved in SNOMED CT development work from early on.

The research team outlined the main advantages of SNOMED CT in our review, despite the fact that other studies have classified the potential advantages of the technology. Our goal in doing this was to outline the particular advantages of using SNOMED CT in conjunction with EHRs. The intention is to draw attention to the fact that additional testing using different data is necessary to determine the validity of the categorization used in this study. It was not established that the set of categories our research team used was exhaustive or comprehensive.

Thus, carefully assessing SNOMED CT use cases from the standpoint of typical benefits may prove relevant in future research. It might also be crucial to investigate the kinds of drawbacks, hazards, and bottlenecks that are discernible. By evaluating different use cases, it might be possible to extract the general success factors of clinical SNOMED CT implementation. Overall, the evaluation of SNOMED CT implementation requires more attention. As an example, the European large-scale implementation of SNOMED CT, which is being funded by the European Commission, could at the same time advance evaluation studies or require systematic evaluation as a part of the funding process.

Based on our review, we found that most articles did a poor job of describing the EHR system or related software, and that there was a lack of a consistent structure for specific EHR descriptions, which resulted in a disorganized collection of information. Since SNOMED CT is meant to facilitate the use of EHRs, this is obviously a problem that needs to be addressed more in future use-case descriptions. If the research's goal is to improve the clinical implementation process by averting potential pitfalls and roadblocks in the past, then describing the capabilities and overall maturity of the EHR system is essential information to include in use case descriptions. We recognize that addressing potential mistakes does not mean that specific implementation experiences are universally generalizable, but that such implementation is required to be adapted to other clinical contexts. To promote the scalability of previous experiences, we suggest, for example, the application of the electronic medical record maturity model (EMRAM) in future use cases.

EMRAM is a widely used tool developed by the Healthcare Information and Management Systems Society to measure the rate of adoption of EHR functions in health care settings. Its stages match the technological progress of the overall digitalization of the health care setting. Moreover, one possible starting point for future studies is to recognize specific use cases for software applications in clinical specialties, in which SNOMED CT would be valuable to accelerate and facilitate specific types of clinical implementations.

Limitations

There are several issues with this systematic review that may compromise the validity of the findings. Our systematic review's procedures and outcomes are openly and thoroughly documented, enabling readers to judge the reliability and relevance of our conclusions. The different levels of description in the research articles proved to be difficult, despite the fact that the methodological foundation of the review is supported by science. For instance, the descriptions of background variables resulted in some degree of imprecision in the results. This especially affected the categories regarding the clinical context and type of EHR. The study's risk of bias was carefully considered during the research process, and no assumptions were made about missing or unclear information from the studies. By doing an extensive and in-depth literature search, we hoped to minimize bias and prevent missing important research. But the results of our search turned up just one database. However, recent research suggests that can serve as the primary search system. PubMed satisfies all performance requirements, including query formulation, query interpretation by the system, and search reproducibility, making it an excellent choice for evidence synthesis in the form of systematic reviews. However, it is impossible to guarantee that a system that has performed well in one set of tests won't perform poorly in another. Moreover, not all SNOMED CT implementation projects are published in the scientific literature. Thus, it is important to recognize that relevant information on clinical use cases may be found in different types of literature.

By summarizing key findings based on evidence-based results, this literature review shows that systematic reviews are pertinent to the advancement of knowledge regarding the use of SNOMED CT and its potential advantages in further facilitating multi-professional, clinically driven implementations. In order to support the scalability of review results, clinical use cases are required. More focus should be placed on describing contextual factors, such as the use of prior frameworks and the electronic health care system currently in use, in order to achieve the best out-of-use case reports and enable results comparability. Regarding future research, although other systematic reviews have addressed similar questions to ours, this review is necessary to shift the focus onto more clinically grounded implementation outcomes and benefits of the use of SNOMED CT. Generally, further research evidence is still needed to determine how exactly SNOMED CT benefits clinical care and patient information quality.

SNOMED CT to ICD-10-CM Map

The world's most comprehensive and multilingual clinical healthcare terminology is SNOMED CT. It is intended to be used in the Electronic Health Record (EHR) for clinical documentation. The SNOMED CT to ICD-10-CM map (also known as "the Map") is designed to facilitate the semi-automated generation of ICD-10-CM codes for statistical and reimbursement purposes from clinical data encoded in SNOMED CT.

The Map can be used in the following scenarios:

- **Real-time use by the healthcare provider** - In this case, the doctor or other healthcare provider uses the EHR's problem list application, which includes the Map. The physician updates the SNOMED CT-encoded problem list at the conclusion of a clinic visit. Utilizing patient context (such as age and gender) and co-morbidities (other problems on the problem list), the Map-enabled problem list application generates a list of ICD-10-CM codes based on algorithmic evaluation of map rules. This process determines the most appropriate candidate ICD-10-CM codes in accordance with ICD-10-CM coding guidelines and conventions. If necessary, the clinician is prompted for additional information to decide between alternative codes, or to refine the output codes. The clinician confirms the suggested ICD-10-CM codes.

- **Retrospective coding by coding professionals** - In this case, coding experts are given candidate ICD-10-CM codes to consider by means of an application that uses the Map and a stored SNOMED CT encoded problem list. There are different levels of automation. In situations where automated rule processing is not available, textual advice may be shown.

Mapping Methodology

The mapping approach closely resembles the SNOMED CT to ICD-10 Crossmap Project, an IHTSDO and World Health Organization collaborative project. To ensure quality and lower variability, terminology specialists with training map data in two independent ways. Discordant maps are examined by a third expert, while identical maps produced independently are recognized as final. To discuss challenging and unclear cases, the team meets on a regular basis.

Rule-based Mapping

A one-to-one mapping between a SNOMED CT concept and an ICD-10-CM code is not always feasible due to the variations in granularity, emphasis, and organizing principles between SNOMED CT and ICD-10-CM. This Map takes a consistent approach to addressing this challenge, as did the IHTSDO and WHO when creating the SNOMED CT to ICD-10 rule-based map. The core of "rule-based mapping" is that each potential target code is represented as a "map rule" when choosing between different ICD-10-CM codes. A "map group" is made up of related map rules. Contextual data and co-morbidities are used to determine the prescribed order in which map rules within a map group are evaluated at run-time. Each map group will resolve to at most one ICD-10-CM code. In the event that a SNOMED CT concept requires more than one ICD-10-CM code to fully represent its meaning, the map will consist of multiple map groups.

Scope

It may be possible to map all currently pre-coordinated SNOMED CT concepts to ICD-10-CM. These concepts fall into three hierarchies: clinical findings, events, and situations with explicit context. Based on the CORE Problem List Subset of SNOMED CT, which includes commonly seen problems, and the Convergent Medical Terminology contents donated by Kaiser Permanente, a priority list of clinically important concepts was identified. Every concept in the US Extension that falls under the purview of mapping has been mapped. The availability of resources and user feedback will determine whether the map's coverage is extended to include additional SNOMED CT concepts.

Release Schedule

The Map is updated with each new SNOMED CT US Edition release

(March and September) and includes the annual ICD-10-CM update.

File Path

The SNOMED CT to ICD-10-CM map is released as Refset 6011000124106 | ICD-10-CM extended map reference set (foundation metadata concept)|. The map data are in the file xder2_iisssccRefset_ExtendedMap(Full/Snapshot)_US1000124_YYYY MMDD.txt, which is in the Map folder under Refset in each release type folder.

Name	Date modified	Type	Size
der2_iisssccRefset_ExtendedMapDelta_US1000124_20180901.txt	8/18/2018 3:40 PM	Text Document	5,589 KB
der2_sRefset_SimpleMapDelta_US1000124_20180901.txt	8/18/2018 3:40 PM	Text Document	659 KB

Fig- File path

License Requirements

Users with licenses to use both SNOMED CT and ICD-10-CM may use the Map in accordance with NLM's mapping assumptions. The International Health Terminology Standards Development Organization (IHTSDO) is the owner of SNOMED CT. As the official U.S. member of the IHTSDO, the NLM disseminates SNOMED CT at no cost in compliance with the rights and obligations of members specified in the IHTSDO's Articles. The License for Use of the UMLS Metathesaurus incorporates the license terms. SNOMED CT may be used freely in IHTSDO Member territories, such as the United States, low-income nations, and for qualifying research projects in any nation, subject to the terms of the IHTSDO Affiliate license.

Omaha System

A taxonomy (classification) based on research, the Omaha System aims to improve information management, documentation, and practice in a variety of contexts. The Omaha System may be used by

HIM professionals in home care, hospice, assisted living and long-term care, public health, schools, hospitals treating chronic illnesses, and other case-management settings.Occupational therapists, physical therapists, registered dieticians, recreational therapists, speech and language pathologists, nurses, doctors, and social workers are among the users.Multidisciplinary health teams have an efficient foundation for documentation, communication, care coordination, and outcome measurement when they apply the Omaha System correctly and consistently.

The Omaha System consists of three components that offer a relational, reliable, and valid structure and set of terms that can link clinical data to demographic, financial, administrative, and staffing data.

Components	Terms	Purpose
Problem Classification Scheme	• 4 domains • 42 problems • 2 sets of modifiers • Clusters of problem specific signs/symptoms	Organize assessment (needs and strengths) for individuals, families, and communities
Intervention Scheme	• 4 categories • 75 targets and 1 other • Client-specific information	Organize multidisciplinary practitioners' care plans and the services they deliver
Problem	• 3 concepts	Evaluate

Rating Scale for Outcomes	• 5-point Likert-type scale	individual, family, or community change over time

Bringing IT to Bear on Key HIM Functions

More and more entries in modern EHRs are composed of structured text meant to facilitate interoperability—the capacity for computerized documentation systems to exchange coded data. Instead of being buried in data cemeteries like file folders or storage media, structured clinical data can be mined to produce insightful research and reports. An EHR system should ideally be made to make it easier to collect data that supports these various, later uses.

Learning about the Omaha System brings new insights and a fresh perspective to documentation processes that can lead to improved data capture and require less intensive efforts by HIM professionals to extract meaningful data. Focusing attention on information management that enhances practitioner workflow and supports quality data capture is the foundation for a well-designed EHR and is a shared value of the Omaha System.

One of the main goals of Lawrence Weed's problem-oriented medical record is to improve the structure and content of progress notes while managing the complexity of clinical data and medical knowledge. The idea behind the problem list was to serve as a focal point for clinicians to keep track of a patient's medical issues in the medical record in a clear and organized manner, as well as to support a systematic approach to problem solving and clinical judgment.

The Omaha System helps clinicians build upon these concepts by focusing attention on the patient problems, supporting a description of the care provided, and then offering a quantifiable method to rate the outcomes achieved.

Capturing Data for Automated Reuse

Technology facilitates communication by using data-mapping tools and embedded clinical terminology standards to automate the multidisciplinary problem list. For instance, mapping enables data to be entered into the EHR using the terminology most appropriate for a healthcare professional's needs after a problem list has been created. The automated data reuse that results helps the researcher or clinician use the data for several more uses.

Mapping creates connections between concepts (such as terminology or classifications) in one data set and the same or strikingly similar concepts in another data set. A healthcare organization's or other providers' ability to share problem lists is facilitated by the use of standard clinical terminology. Additionally, the mapping makes it possible to connect issues with their solutions and facilitates the examination of how those interventions relate to results.

Controlled vocabularies, mapping, and data content standards have numerous advantages. The reporting of laboratory data, the use of order sets, clinical guidelines, clinical system alerts and reminders, and the automated retrieval of pertinent medical literature within an EHR are all made easier by consistent, standardized term naming. Practitioners can objectively concentrate on pertinent information at the point of care by using a classification system like the Omaha System. In practice, education, and research settings, the Omaha System assists in recording and assessing various aspects of care, such as issues, solutions, and results.

The Problem-Solving Process

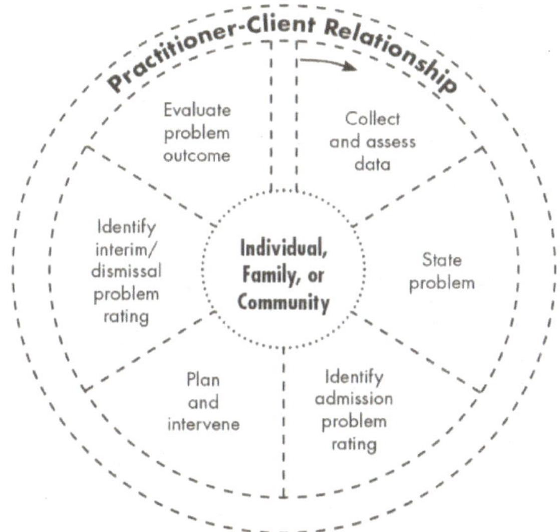

Fig- Relationship between practitioner and clients

The relationship between the practitioner and the client, as well as the ideas of clinical decision-making, quality improvement, and critical thinking, are all incorporated into the Omaha System model. The problem-solving process is also dynamic, interactive, and circular.The partnership with multidisciplinary practitioners and the crucial roles of the individual, family, and community are identified at the center of the model.

Describing the System: Components and Terms

The Problem Classification Scheme, the Intervention Scheme, and the Problem Rating Scale for Outcomes are the three parts of the Omaha System (refer to "Omaha System Overview" on page 45). The constituents provide users with a valid, dependable, and relational structure and vocabulary that facilitates the integration of clinical data with administrative, financial, demographic, and staffing data.

The circular, interactive nature of the process from data collection, critical thinking, and clinical decision making through to evaluation and quality improvement is reflected in the system model (above). The dynamics of the practitioner-client relationship are where this process takes place. The partnership with multidisciplinary practitioners and the crucial roles of the individual, family, and community are identified at the center of the model.

"Collect and assess data" and "state problem," the two leading wedges of the model's circle, are equivalent to the Problem Classification Scheme. The system is a thorough, systematic, non-exhaustive, mutually exclusive taxonomy intended to recognize a variety of health-related issues. Four levels of assessment are arranged using its straightforward language, ranging from general to specific. The wedge "plan and intervene" is equivalent to the Intervention Scheme. Its structure is hierarchical and resembles the Problem Classification Scheme. Multidisciplinary health professionals use it to describe care plans and services; its three levels of actions or activities flow from general to specific.

The Problem Rating Scale for Outcomes is equivalent to three wedges: "identify admission problem rating," "identify interim/dismissal problem rating," and "evaluate problem outcome." It measures the entire range of severity for the concepts of knowledge, behavior, and status. Each subscale provides a continuum for examining problem-specific ratings for individuals, families, or communities at regular or predictable times.

Years in the Making, Use Increasing

The Omaha System was created by practitioners as a result of four federally supported study initiatives carried out between 1975 and 1993. Revisions and refinements were made to the structure and terminology, and reliability, validity, and usability were established by staff and managers at the Visiting Nurse Association of Omaha and seven other test sites. The Omaha System was designed to be as simple, quick, and adaptable as it could be. Its definitions, codes, structure, and terms are all free to use without restriction because they are not protected by copyright. The Omaha System is in the public domain, but publications and software must identify a reference to it in order to preserve its integrity.

The Omaha System was first implemented in US community settings. Use has increased both internationally and throughout the care continuum. At 300 sites, about 8,000 practitioners use the Omaha System point-of-care software, while 2,000 practitioners keep paper records. Vendors who use the Omaha System as the foundation for their clinical documentation software are becoming more and more numerous. One of the earliest terms recognized by the American Nurses Association in 1992 was the Omaha System. It is recognized by the standards body Health Level Seven and integrated into SNOMED CT, LOINC, and the National Library of Medicine's Metathesaurus. It is also indexed in CINAHL. The Omaha System met the tier 2 selection criteria for a use case in the Healthcare Information Technology Standards Panel in 2007.

Teaching through Case Studies

The case of Ander M., which is discussed on the ensuing pages, highlights the importance of using standardized terminology when describing the treatments and care requirements. The case study is divided into two sections: an explanation and solutions.The narrative describes the services that a home care nurse provided to a fictitious client named Ander M. Referral information, information the nurse collected during the visit, hints for identifying Omaha System issues, ratings, and interventions are all included.Terms from the Problem Rating Scale for Outcomes, the Intervention Scheme, and the Problem Classification Scheme are used in the answers. Select answers are clarified by succinct remarks enclosed in parenthesis.

Promoting Good Documentation at the Time of Care

One crucial task performed by HIM specialists is the review of documentation after it has been created. The Omaha System makes quality documentation easier to create, which benefits patients at the point of care. Better care is the outcome of using the Omaha System, which can affect data integrity and documentation quality. HIM specialists can gain from knowing how the system smoothly integrates patient care with data integrity. Utilizing a multitude of potential health IT benefits, such as developing outcomes data, supporting evidence-based practice, and incorporating data standards and terminologies, the system fosters innovation.

Chapter - 7

e-Health: Patients & the Internet

Use of Information & Communication Technologies to Support Effective Work Practice Innovation in the Health Sector

Adopting information and communication technologies (ICT) widely is a crucial tactic to address the issues that global health systems face, including rising costs, shrinking resources, and a shortage of workers. ICT investment has increased quickly, but adoption and acceptance have lagged, and the benefits have not been as great as anticipated. A multi-site investigation of how ICT can promote and drive innovative work practices has been missing from the research literature. This project, which is based in Australia, will evaluate the conditions under which health service organizations can use ICT and the degree to which these systems encourage the development of new, long-term service delivery models that boost capacity and offer quick, secure, efficient, economical, and long-lasting medical care.

In addition to developing and testing new ICT use models that support innovations in work practices, a multi-method approach will be used to measure the current impact of ICT on workforce practices. Three widely used commercial ICT systems—computerized ordering systems, ambulatory electronic medical record systems, and emergency medicine information systems—will be the subject of the study. These systems are being adopted in Australia and other nations. The five main characteristics of work practice innovation that we will assess and evaluate are: modifications to the roles and duties of professionals; incorporation of best practices into routine care; safe care practices; team-based care delivery; and active consumer involvement in care.

The workforce and organizational complexity of the health sector will be examined and interpreted using a socio-technical approach to ICT use. The project will also highlight ICT as a potentially disruptive innovation that could upend current models of care delivery and, as a result, cause some health professionals to see it as a threat to established roles and responsibilities. These opinions have suppressed discussion and prevented broader investigations of ICT's possible advantages; however, there is little concrete proof that role modifications affect health care outcomes. This project will provide important evidence about the role of ICT insupporting new models of care delivery across multiple healthcare organizations and about the ways in which innovative work practice change is diffused.

Global health systems are under pressure to provide more complex services, but they are constrained by budget and are expected to experience a shortage of medical personnel in the near future. The aging of the population, the need for more complex care, and the advancement of medical technology are all driving up healthcare delivery costs in OECD countries. In Australia, for example, health is already one of the most expensive sectors of the economy, at 9.3% of GDP by 2045 this allocation is predicted to rise to at least 16% One of the single most important challenges for health systems, then, is to establish new models of service delivery which increase capacity and provide rapid, safe, effective and affordable health care, and do so sustainably, within health workforce and resource constraints. A key strategy being advanced to meet this challenge is increased use of information and communication technologies (ICT).

The desire to improve work practices, service outcomes, and productivity has led to over $US3.5 trillion in global expenditure on ICT across all sectors. Developed health systems like those in the US, Canada, and Australia are investing more in ICT as a means of achieving the improvements in service outcomes and productivity that are visible in other industries.

According to studies, ICT use in the health sector can improve integration of best practices into routine care, increase efficiency, decrease errors, support more team-based care, empower patients to take a more active role in their care, and result in more efficient services by altering professional roles and responsibilities. This has only, however, been proven in exemplary organizations and singular projects. There is insufficient proof of significant adjustments in work practices that are backed by ICT use. According to available data, ICT investment has increased quickly, but uptake has been sluggish and benefits have not been as great as anticipated. There have also been instances where ICT has had unanticipated, detrimental effects on safety and efficiency.

The health sector has had only patchy success implementing ICT using strategies that are employed in other industries. This can be partially attributed to the distinct organizational and workforce features within the industry. Healthcare institutions are intricately designed. The main professional groups function in hierarchical structures, exhibit high degrees of autonomy, and exhibit tribal behaviors. The nature of work is highly specialized and non-linear. However, horizontal work coordination is necessary for safe and productive work, especially when there are strong professional group collaborations. For this reason, effective interprofessional and organizational communication is essential.

Furthermore, rather than making complex tasks simpler or eliminating them entirely, ICT in the health sector appears to increase intellectual content and complexity of work, in contrast to certain other industries. On the other hand, the business process reengineering methods for changing work practices that have been popular in health information and communication technology (ICT) projects are typically founded on top-down linear workflow models and are frequently insufficient to handle the intricate collaborative nature of medical work. The high number of large-scale health IT project failures that have been reported demonstrates the limitations of these traditional approaches to ICT work practice reform.

Constant changes in the systems used cause additional problems. For example, a survey of over 800 participants at an annual electronic medical record (EMR) trade fair in the US in 2007 found that 19% of respondents reported that they had or were in the process of de-installing an EMR system.

The quest for methods that emphasize the connections between the technical (tools, hardware, equipment, and processes) and social (people, values, norms, and culture) facets of organizations has resulted from these failures. Studies on Computer-Supported Cooperative Work (CSCW), for instance, have looked into how people work in groups and individually with devices like flight simulators. However, a drawback of research on human-technology interaction is that it mostly rests on a theory of command and control. For instance, a small team follows clear guidelines while performing a series of tasks in the cockpit. This is a comparatively quiet and well-defined workplace. Research on such limited organizational structures has dubious applicability to more complex and dispersed work environments. The health sector, with its many professional subgroups, complex work processes and power structures, represents a much more fluid and dynamic context with fewer formalised control mechanisms.

Gaps in knowledge

The health sector lacks research-based, empirically-tested models for implementing significant changes in work processes and structures in order to fully reap the benefits of information and communication technology. Rather, short-term, single-site studies that are mainly descriptive have dominated global research in this field. Additionally, researchers have devoted nearly all of their attention to examining companies that have created their own ICT systems. Almost 25% of the studies in a systematic review on the effects of ICT use in health were carried out in one of four US medical centers, all of which had in-house systems.

Out of 257 studies, only 9 percent looked at commercial systems. However, a large majority of organizations in Australia, as in other nations, use commercial systems. Since the majority of these systems were created in the US, they may not work well in other health jurisdictions because they were created for American health delivery models. Because of this, they pose unique difficulties for health systems that are primarily supported by public funding and may make it more difficult to use them to support changes in work practices. In conclusion, little is known about the reasons behind the notable changes in work practices that certain organizations are able to accomplish, while others utilizing the same ICT systems are unable to. This raises questions about which factors enable or inhibit ICT-supported work innovation. In previous studies we have shown that characteristics of team and organisational cultures are associated with effective ICT use, but there are likely to be other significant factors.

As a result, the evidence supporting and propelling innovative work practice change through ICT is typically weak and primarily derived from case studies of individual organizations that are not broadly applicable. Now, extensive multi-site studies are required. This is essential to create safer health systems as well as the necessary productivity gains. ICT plays a key role in enhancing communication and teamwork to deliver a safer health system. Research has demonstrated that inadequate communication and a lack of teamwork are major causes of the harm that one in ten patients experience as a result of the care they receive.

The aim of this research is to conduct a large-scale, multi-site study to measure current ICT impact on workforce practices. It will also develop and test new models of ICT use which support innovations in work practice.

Methods

The study will be conducted within the Sydney South West Area Health Service (SSWAHS), which serves 1.4 million residents in central and south western Sydney with publicly funded healthcare services. The population is representative of Australia's most ethnically diverse Area Health Service. SSWAHS employs more than 17,000 people and runs and oversees 17 healthcare organizations.

Interventions

This study will concentrate on three information and communication technologies: emergency medicine information systems, ambulatory electronic medical record systems, and computerized ordering systems. There are plenty of opportunities for work innovation in all three of the ICT interventions.

Data collection methods

We will conduct in-person observations of practice across a number of locations in order to spot innovations and shifts in work roles. Interviews and video observation will go along with this. These data will shed light on how roles and responsibilities have changed, how teams interact, how consumers are involved, and what elements clinicians have found to be supportive of or impeding work innovation. In addition to non-participant observation of project steering and organizational committees, the data will be integrated with analyses of organizational documents. System functionality evaluations will be undertaken in conjunction with user feedback (via surveys, observations and interviews) about system performance, specifically in relation to integration of ICT with work practices. Observational studies and interviews will focus on identification of workaround procedures, as we have foundthese are often introduced to accommodate systems which fail to integrate with work practices, or where practices have not been changed to take advantage of work process efficiencies which ICT offer.

We will use our expertise in social network analyses to look at social and communication networks. We will concentrate on work task areas that have been recognized as opportunities for work innovation, building on our previous findings. The social network analyses will look at how connected participants are among the enrolled organizations and how discussions and ideas about changing work practices are shared within and between departments, services, and discipline areas. Additionally, the social network analyses will look into and offer an assessment of team-based care. This will be quantified further using the Team Climate Inventory (TCI), a tool to gauge the extent of team cohesiveness and innovation. We have shown that teams with high TCI scores report more innovative use of ICT. The Organisational Culture Inventory (OCI), which we have demonstrated is able to discriminate between cultures in health organisations, will also be administered.

Through the development and validation of our Work Observation Method by Activity Timing (WOMBAT), we will be able to compute quantitative changes in the work patterns of clinicians. Individuals are directly observed in a structured manner using this method. Using a personal digital assistant (PDA), the observer logs details about what, with whom, and how each task is completed as well as interruptions and multitasking. Work patterns can be quantified since the PDA automatically timestamps tasks.

We will measure the effects of ICT-supported work innovation using a range of indicators including changes in:

organisational productivity measures such as number of patients treated and tests processed, lengths of patients' stays in hospitals, emergency department and outpatient visit length, and staffing levels and mix;effectiveness and safety indicators such as changes in rates of medication error and unnecessary duplicate test orders; andefficiency indicators such as turnaround time of test results, and staff time consumed by specific categories of work.

To calculate the cost-effectiveness of ICT-supported work innovations, these data will be measured and paired with system implementation and maintenance expenses. We will make use of costing data from earlier studies as well as local financial data. Results will be put to the test by asking stakeholder groups for input as they become available. In order to actively participate in the process of interpreting data and forming the research conclusions, staff members at the participating sites will be recruited.

Exemplar sub-studies

An electronic toxic drug monitoring system (eTDMS) has been developed as part of the rheumatology ambulatory electronic medical record (eMR) to help clinicians monitor patients with rheumatology who are prescribed toxic drugs, also known as Disease Modifying Anti-rheumatic Drugs (DMARDs). This sub-study aims to assess how well the eTDMS works in terms of appropriate drug monitoring, how long it takes nursing staff to monitor patients, and how it affects clinicians' work processes. The first part of this study will use a before and after study design to assess whether using the eMR has improved toxic drug monitoring. The sample size for this sub-study, based on power of 80% to detect a difference between pre and post intervention sample proportions at p = 0.05 is 60 patients in each study period. Work process changes will be identified using work process maps, interviews with clinicians, and time and motion work measurement studies of nurses in the clinic. The intervention will then be trialled at a second rheumatology clinic in another hospital and results of that trial compared.

Emergency medicine clinical information systems

In the emergency departments (EDs) of eight hospitals, a cross-sectional qualitative study utilizing focus groups, interviews, observation, and video ethnography will be carried out. Every method will be aimed at gathering data regarding the opinions and methods of clinicians regarding the ICT systems they employ, how they have altered routine work procedures, and the particular impacts they have on roles within the profession, communication, and patient outcomes. There will be focus groups and interviews with a sample of about 100 clinical staff members. Further, a social network analysis to measure the ways in which senior emergency clinicians are connected across the eight hospitals will be conducted and the extent to which social networks influence the diffusion of new work practices with ICT assessed. This will involve a sample of approximately 70 senior emergency clinicians from across the eight hospitals.

The Sydney South West Area Health Service Human Research Ethics Committee Multi-center project No.09/CRGH/53, CH62/6/2009-046 gave ethics approval for the entire study. This includes giving informed consent when participants demand it.

We will approach the use of ICT in health from a socio-technical perspective. This will get around some of the drawbacks of earlier methods and offer a strong theoretical framework for analyzing and interpreting the organizational and workforce complexities of the health sector. In the proposed project, we will expand on this conceptual work by investigating the role of ICT as a possible disruptive innovation. This phrase describes technological advancements that put the status quo to the test and frequently overturn it. While industry incumbents perceive these technologies as threatening, consumers frequently embrace them.

For example, commentators external to the health sector have argued that such technologies are needed in health in order to change traditional patterns of work and "enable less expensive professionals to do progressively more sophisticated things in less expensive settings". Professional bodies, on the other hand, have voiced concerns about possible role changes. The limited evidence as to the effects of role changes on service outcomes continues to stifle discussion as well as wider explorations of how ICT can be used to provide more efficient health services. Our research will provide important evidence to inform this debate and provide the evidence-base for relevant health policy.

Evidence of the diffusion of innovative work practices is a planned outcome of this research. Research already conducted shows that communication patterns both within and between organizations have an impact on the uptake and dissemination of new concepts and innovations. Research conducted outside of the health field has demonstrated that the most innovative organizations have cultures that promote teamwork, open communication, and the generation of new ideas. Drawing upon uncertainty reduction theory which argues that individuals communicate in order to reduce uncertainty and that this process ties people together and promotes further interactions, Albrecht studied three large organizations and found that staff were most likely to report the embracing of new ideas if discussion about work and social matters also occurred. The proposed research, unlike previous single-site studies, will have the capacity to examine the ways in which innovative work practices and ideas are distributed within and across communities and organizations within an area health service.

This project, which is based in Australia, will tackle a major issue facing the global health sector: how to use ICT to develop new and improved service delivery models that boost capacity and offer quick, safe, efficient, and reasonably priced medical care while maintaining sustainability and working within the limitations of the health workforce and resources. The project will create and evaluate new implementation models in addition to measuring the present impact of ICT on workforce practices. By investigating the ways in which ICT can support work innovation to achieve new models of health service delivery that result in quantifiable improvements, this research will add to the body of knowledge in the field of health informatics. It will also track the dissemination of innovative practices.

Public Health Informatics

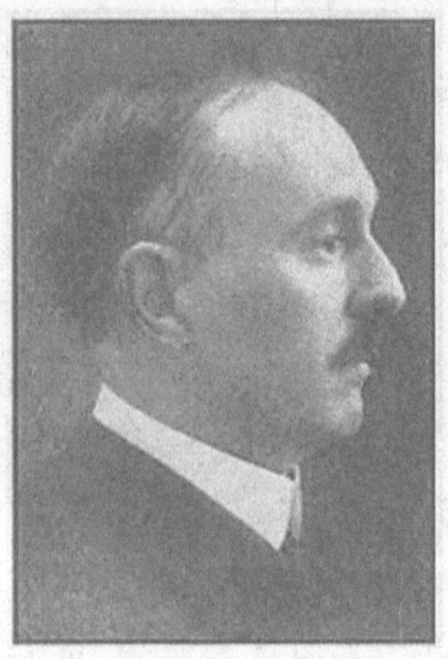

Public health informatics is the systematic application of information and computer science and technology to public health practice, research, and learning.

The science and art of preventing disease, prolonging life, and promoting health through the organized efforts and informed choices of society, organizations, public and private communities, and individuals." — CEA Winslow Information science Theories in information science try to explain how we think, store, retrieve, and transmit information.

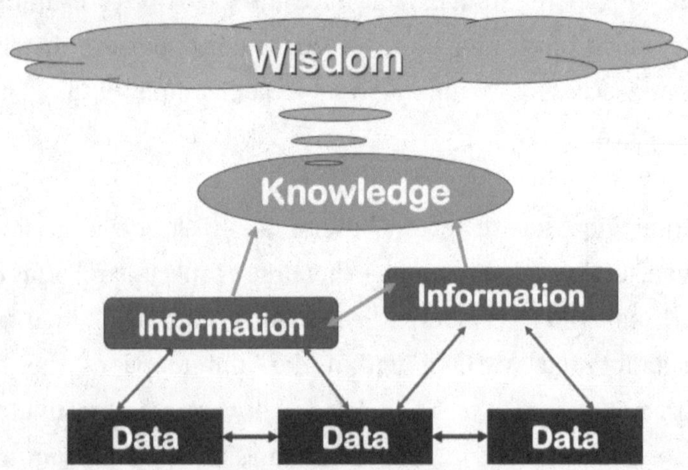

Integrating Informatics Principles in Public Health

Data = undigested observations and unvarnished facts ...

- Fact, text, graphic, image, sound ...
- Without meaningful relation to anything else ...
- A thing

Information = organized data ...

• Formatted, filtered, organized, structured, interpreted, summarized data ...

• data + meaning = information ...

• Relates to a description, definition or perspective (what, who, when , where)

The Mission of Public Health

Satisfying the desire of society to provide environments conducive to human health. —Medicine Institute. "The goal of public health is to benefit the greatest number of people possible." —Global Health OrganizationClinical care, sometimes referred to as health care, is the prevention, management, and treatment of disease as well as the maintenance of physical and mental well-being through the services provided by the medical and allied health professions.

Determinant: Element that plays a role in the development of a trait. Epidemics or outbreaks are defined as the occurrence of a disease, a particular health-related behavior, or any other health-related event that is manifestly more common than expected in a community or region. Although the terms can be used interchangeably, epidemic typically denotes a more widespread geographic spread of disease or health-related incidents.

The use of computers, clinical guidelines, communication, and information systems is known as public health informatics, and it encompasses the vast majority of public health and related professions, including nursing, clinical and hospital care, public health, and medical research.Public health informatics is practiced by people working in federal, state, and larger local health jurisdictions as well as public health agencies in developed nations such as the United States. Furthermore, numerous academic institutions conduct public health informatics research and provide training.

At the federal Centers for Disease Control and Prevention in US states like Atlanta, Georgia, the Public Health Surveillance and Informatics Program Office (PHSIPO) focuses on advancing the state of information science and applies digital information technologies to aid in the detection and management of diseases and syndromes in individuals and populations.

The bulk of the work of public health informatics in the United States, as with public health generally, takes place at the state and local level, in the state departments of health and the county or parish departments of health. At a state health department the activities may include: collection and storage of *vital statistics* (birth and death records); collection of reports of communicable disease cases from doctors, hospitals, and laboratories, used for infectious disease surveillance; display of infectious disease statistics and trends; collection of child immunization and lead screening information; daily collection and analysis of emergency room data to detect early evidence of biological threats; collection of hospital capacity information to allow for planning of responses in case of emergencies. Each of these activities presents its own information processing challenge.

Collection of public health data

Public health organizations with adequate IT resources have been moving toward web-based public health data collection since the early days of the World Wide Web. More recently, these agencies have also been utilizing automated messaging systems to disseminate the same data. Approximately between 2000 and 2005, the National Electronic Disease Surveillance System (NEDSS) of the Centers for Disease Control and Prevention developed and made available to states at no cost a comprehensive web-based and message-based reporting system known as the NEDSS Base System (NBS).

Only a few states and larger counties have developed their own versions of electronic disease surveillance systems, such as Pennsylvania's PA-NEDSS, due to funding constraints and the unsoundness of fiefdom-based systems. In comparison to the NEDSS federal product, these do not offer full intestate notification services in a timely manner, which raises disease rates.

The CDC has promoted the use of various industry-standard messaging formats and vocabularies in public health data exchange in order to foster interoperability. The most well-known of these are the Systematized Nomenclature of Medicine (SNOMED) vocabulary of health care concepts, the LOINC system for encoding laboratory test and result information, and the Health Level 7 (HL7) standards for health care messaging.

The Public Health Information Network is an idea that the CDC has been pushing since around 2005. Its purpose is to make it easier for data from various partners in the health care industry and beyond (hospitals, clinical and environmental laboratories, physician practices, pharmacies) to be transmitted to local health agencies, state health agencies, and ultimately the CDC. The entity must be able to receive the data, store it, aggregate it properly, and transmit it to the next level at each stage. An example would be the legal requirement for hospitals, labs, and physicians to report infectious disease data to local health agencies, which in turn must report to the state public health department. States are also required to report the data to the CDC in aggregate form. Among other uses, the CDC publishes the Morbidity and Mortality Weekly Report (MMWR) based on these data acquired systematically from across the United States.

The following are the main problems with gathering public health data: variations in reporting requirements among states, territories, and localities; lack of resources for both the reporter and the collector; and incompatibility of data interchange formats, which can be at the purely syntactic or semantic level.

⇨ Public health informatics can be thought or divided into three categories.

i. Study models of different systems

Finding and studying models of complex systems, like the spread of disease, falls under the first category. This can be accomplished through a variety of data collection methods, including electronic surveys submitted to the organization (like the CDC) or surveys conducted in hospitals. You can find out about disease incidence, transmission rates, and surveillance by contacting international organizations like WHO or government agencies like the CDC. Examining disease transmission/rates is not the only option. Additionally, public health informatics can investigate the rates at which individuals visit doctors and whether they have health insurance or not. Before the advent of the internet, public health data in the United States, like other healthcare and business data, were collected on paper forms and stored centrally at the relevant public health agency. If the data were to be computerized they required a distinct data entry process, were stored in the various file formats of the day and analyzed by mainframe computers using standard batch processing.

ii. Storage of public health data

The second area of focus is how to make various public health systems more efficient. This is accomplished through a variety of data collection techniques, data storage, and data application to address contemporary health issues. All systems must use the same vocabulary and word usage in order to maintain standardization. To keep everything current, it's critical to discover new methods for systems to communicate with one another and exchange new data. The data management problems that other industries face are also present in the storage of public health data. And just like in other sectors, the type of data being managed has an impact on how these problems manifest in specifics.

Data modeling is particularly difficult because public health data, like data on health care in general, is complex and variable. A generation ago, it was common practice to use flat data sets for statistical analysis; however, modern public health enterprises demand more sophistication due to interoperability requirements and integrated data sets. Informatics for public health is increasingly using relational databases. Achieving a feasible balance between intricate and abstract data models, like the CDC's Public Health Logical Data Model or HL7's Information Model (RIM), and more basic, impromptu models that even inexperienced public health practitioners can create and utilize is a challenge for designers and implementers of the numerous data sets needed for diverse public health applications.

Due to the variability of the incoming data to public health jurisdictions, data quality assurance is also a major issue.

iii. Analysis of public health data

The last category, which is maintaining and improving current models and systems to handle the flood of data, can be conceptualized as the storing and sorting of this new data. This can be as easy as making a direct connection to an electronic data collection source, like hospital health records, or it can involve accessing public data (CDC) regarding disease rates and transmission. Developing new algorithms that can efficiently and rapidly sift through massive amounts of data is also essential.

The public health informaticist must become proficient with a variety of analysis tools in order to extract useful public health information from the vast amount of data that is currently available. These tools include business intelligence tools for creating regular or ad hoc reports, sophisticated statistical analysis tools like DAP/SAS and PSPP/SPSS, and Geographic Information Systems (GIS) for revealing the geographic aspect of public health trends. Such analyses typically call for techniques that adequately protect the confidentiality of the medical records. Sorting the data into individually identifiable variables and discarding the rest is one method.

Applications in health surveillance and epidemiology

Professionals who wish to get more involved in public health informatics can find helpful information from a few organizations. The American Medical Informatics Association (AMIA) is a professional association for those working in the fields of biomedical research, informatics, and health care. This includes researchers, scientists, physicians, and students. AMIA's primary objectives are to advance the field of public health informatics, assist in enhancing the impact of health innovations, and go from "bench to bedside." They provide free webinars, online courses, and annual conferences to their members. Additionally, there is a career center dedicated to the field of biomedical and health informatics.

Role of Nurse in Informatics

Over the past few decades, healthcare technology has made incredible strides that have provided medical professionals with more reliable and abundant data than ever before. Additionally, as informatics has advanced, nurses can now use the data produced by these scientific marvels to give patients better care and treatment. Numerous advancements in the delivery of healthcare, such as the adoption of digital health records, the standardization of diagnostic data, the simplification of the administration of health insurance, and the enhancement of patient privacy, have been made possible by informatics. Nursing informatics, a subfield of health informatics, applies information technology and data management techniques to enhance patient care procedures and avoid unfavorable health outcomes.

The bulk of direct care practitioners are nurses, which puts them in a unique position to have an impact as specialized experts at the nexus of healthcare and technology. In today's healthcare system, registered nurses play roles in operations, education, leadership, and technology in addition to clinical care. Through the use of nursing informatics, nurses can provide patient-centered, evidence-based care, enhance human health, and progress medical research. Additionally, it improves clinical workflows, enabling nurses and other staff to provide patients with more effective and efficient care.

The History of Nursing Informatics in Healthcare

Despite the fact that nursing informatics is becoming a crucial part of healthcare delivery, creative nurses have long used data to enhance patient care and clinical practice. In order to improve sanitation through nursing and medical protocols, Florence Nightingale, a pioneer in the field of healthcare, began gathering, organizing, and processing data in the 1850s, which is when nursing informatics first emerged. Information technology use specifically for nurses began in the 1960s, slightly over a century later.

The first nursing and computer conference was held in the ensuing ten years, and American and British healthcare professionals published nursing-specific informatics papers internationally. Next, we witnessed developments like the formation of the International Medical Informatics Association (IMIA) Nursing Informatics working group and the International Council of Nurses (ICN) practice-related initiatives in the 1980s and early 1990s. In 1983, the U.S. newsletter Computers in Nursing was established. It served as the precursor to the journal CIN: Computers, Informatics, Nursing.

In 1992, the American Nurses Association officially recognized and defined nursing informatics as a specialty practice. Simultaneously, the field's official certification program was established. Since then, in order to stay up to date with the rapidly changing fields of theory, practice, and technology, updates have been made to both the core curriculum and certification requirements. Additionally, organized initiatives have been made to promote workforce training and informatics education. The TIGER (Technology Informatics Guiding Education Reform) Initiative, which was launched in 2006, is one of the most prominent examples.

The Benefits of Nursing Informatics

Through the driving force behind the application of critical healthcare technologies, nursing informatics has reduced the risk of unfavorable outcomes by revolutionizing patient care and improving patient safety. Electronic medical records, or EMRs, for example, allow healthcare professionals, such as nurses, to store patients' entire medical history digitally. This allows them to track patient data over time, identify patients who should be scheduled for checkups or preventive screenings, keep track of how well patients are doing on health parameters like blood pressure and vaccinations, and assess and improve the overall quality of care provided by a practice.

Electronic health records (EMRs) offer even greater benefits, allowing physicians and nurses to perform all of the functions that EMRs do plus much more. They focus on each patient's overall health rather than just standard clinical data. In order to ensure coordinated, patient-focused care, they are therefore made to be shared among all of the patient's healthcare providers, including doctors, nurses, laboratory technicians, specialists, and others. As a result, they contain data gathered by each of these experts. With the use of electronic health records (EHRs), a patient's primary care physician can obtain information about a patient's specific life-threatening allergy, for example, which allows the emergency department clinician to make necessary adjustments to the patient's care—even if the patient is unconscious. In order to better structure and organize the specific data found in EHRs and enable prompt identification and treatment of a large number of patients, informatics is also applied to this data. Working with his team, Dr. Matthew Solomon, a researcher at the Kaiser Permanente Division of Research in Oakland, California, and cardiologist at the Permanente Medical Group, created and verified a software technology that could achieve precisely that. They then used it on their database of echocardiograms, which included nearly a million reports from the previous ten years. It would have likely taken years for doctors to manually identify nearly 54,000 patients with valvular heart disease, but the software did so in a matter of minutes. Another benefit of nursing informatics is that a nurse's notes from a patient's hospital stay can be used to create discharge instructions and a plan for follow-up care, allowing the individual to seamlessly transition from one care setting to another.

Additionally, by assisting caregivers in identifying signs of criminal abuse and safeguarding victims, nursing informatics has improved patient safety. The John Peter Smith Hospital in Fort Worth, Texas, employs nurses who created and implemented an algorithm to recognize signs of human trafficking and intimate partner abuse. The algorithm provides step-by-step instructions to the nurses in the emergency department (ED), integrates seamlessly and effectively with their workflow, and contains a narrative for use in the unlikely event that the patient is found to be a victim. Patients are then given immediate assistance.

By using technology to make it easier to gather, analyze, and report on better quality data about patient safety concerns and health outcomes—as well as to prevent medical errors and enable better monitoring and reporting of those that do occur—nursing informatics enhances safety. Informatics also makes it possible for people in leadership positions, like CNIOs, to create, develop, and apply decision support tools; train other nurses on how to use them; and use predictive analytics tools to find patients and population groups that are at risk.

Nursing Informatics Careers

Experts at every level are required to gather health data, process findings, and convey conclusions to clinicians and other stakeholders as nursing informatics takes on a more central role in hospitals and other healthcare organizations. Patient care and organizational effectiveness are greatly impacted by nurse informaticists, from front-line practice to executive-level leadership.

Nurse Informaticist

A nurse informaticist, sometimes referred to as an informatics nurse, manages sizable amounts of medical data in order to improve population health and nursing practice. By conducting research on issues impacting patients and caregivers, these nursing professionals contribute significantly to improving care, reducing costs, and boosting efficiency.

In addition to their technical duties, some nurse informaticists also work as clinicians, while others are analysts and consultants. Nurse informaticists make sure that regulations and guidelines like the Food and Drug Administration (FDA) and the Health Insurance Portability and Accountability Act (HIPAA) are followed because security is a major concern in the healthcare industry.

Other job responsibilities might include:

- Determining a healthcare organization's needs and implementing technology that meets those requirements.
- Designing and delivering training on devices and applications to health practitioners and patients.
- Communicating key data findings to stakeholders to promote data-driven decision-making in processes and care plans.

Nursing Informatics Specialist

At the specialist level, a nurse informaticist's job description is largely the same and frequently includes clinical work in addition to technical duties. However, nurses holding this title typically have more specialized skills, more responsibilities, and higher earning potential because the specialist role requires higher education levels.

Perioperative Informatics Nurse

A nurse informaticist with expertise in patient care before, during, and after surgical procedures is known as a perioperative informatics nurse. Typically, this includes the patient's admission to the hospital or doctor's office through their discharge. Additionally, a perioperative informatics nurse contributes to the implementation of expanded and novel models of care, thereby enhancing the perioperative process. They work in clinical settings as well as in the field of health information technology (HIT) research.

Chief Nursing Informatics Officer

Within healthcare organizations, a professional in this role is directly involved in management, leadership, and administration. They lead important initiatives pertaining to the implementation, upkeep, and optimization of health information technology and collaborate with other leaders in the field to develop technological solutions. In strategic conversations with stakeholders like business partners and senior leadership, the CNIO also speaks for the needs of nurses.

This business partnership includes exchanging insights and best practices to enhance internal procedures as well as assessments and suggestions for new technologies. Assessing whether clinical operations successfully satisfy the needs of patients and clinicians and identifying opportunities for innovation and improvement are two more important responsibilities.

The job description of a CNIO also includes:

- Developing and employing health data tools.
- Collecting, analyzing and reporting data related to safety issues and outcomes.
- Developing and overseeing policies and procedures for data analysis.

Become a Nurse Informaticist With the Right Education

Depending on the career path you wish to take, there may be additional educational requirements even though all nurse informatics professionals are registered nurses. For instance, entry-level nurse informaticists typically hold an associate's or bachelor's degree in nursing along with coursework toward a bachelor's degree in a related field, such as data analytics or health information technology. In order to become a specialist in the field, you will require graduate-level training in informatics or a related discipline. Additionally, you will probably need a master's degree in nursing (MSN) or nursing informatics to work as an executive or director in the field. Some candidates even hold a doctorate in nursing, or PhD. These positions are within the reach of registered nurses who are interested in this expanding and crucial field of practice through continued education.

Because patient care and healthcare information technology (HIT) are always changing, working nurses have many opportunities to grow in their careers and broaden their skill sets. Your preparation for success in nursing informatics as a skilled and knowledgeable healthcare provider, HIT professional, and business leader will come from Carlow University's Dual Master of Science in Nursing in Education and Leadership and Master of Business Administration (MSN – MBA) degree program. Advance your career in a flexible online environment that caters to working students. Learn from knowledgeable teachers with practical experience who will give you the same focused attention as students on campus. A friendly, encouraging, and helpful community that supports both professional and personal development is a feature of our program.

Chapter -8

Using Information in Healthcare Management

Nursing Information Systems

The environments in which health care is provided are dynamic, complex, and always changing. Demands for information are rising due to changes in medical treatments, rules governing federal and state reimbursement, and increased public awareness of the importance of making both individual and group health care decisions. Computer systems are being developed to gather, store, retrieve, analyze, and communicate health status and health care information in order to proactively address these changes and the increasing demands for clinical information. When the systems are built using informatics concepts, it can help with data collection, storage, retrieval, and analysis related to patient care activities. Computerized information systems that are properly developed and implemented can convert patient care data into knowledge and information that is both clinically and practically relevant.

One of the biggest consumer-focused industries that stands to gain significantly from computerization is the health sector. Over the past few years, there has been a steady rise in the number of healthcare providers and organizations utilizing information and communication technology to improve the way that healthcare is delivered at various levels, including primary, ambulatory, and tertiary care. Every hospital will eventually need to install a healthcare information system as a result of modernization. These are computer and communication systems that healthcare providers use to gather, process, store, and analyze data. To collect and integrate clinical and financial data, it combines computer and communication technologies.

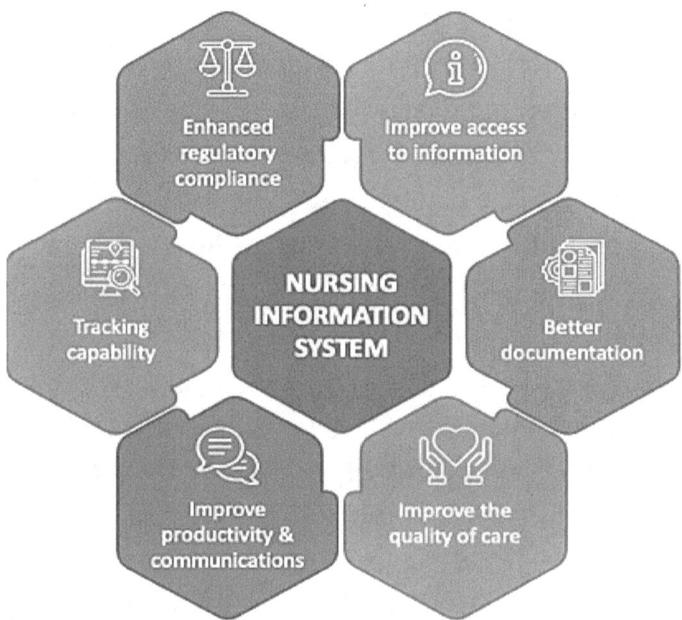

Fig- Nursing information system

Importance of Nursing Information Systems

Information from the clinical sciences (medicine, pharmacy, dentistry, nursing, allied health, and rehabilitation) as well as the management, behavioral, information, and communication sciences can be incorporated into the components of a healthcare information system, enabling clinical and health management decision-making. The field of information sciences in medicine is still expanding, and in recent years, informatics has started to permeate clinical practice more widely. Nonetheless, this field has a very broad scope. Informatics is used in the creation of computer tools for research, in the design of decision supports for practitioners, and in the examination of the body of knowledge that constitutes medicine itself.

The integration of numerous specialized resources in patient care remains a challenge for nurses, given the tremendous advancements in medical science. Access to essential information from these specialized sources frequently limits nursing decisions; hence, prompt and easy access to all relevant patient data is essential. In order to enter the field of information systems, nurses might find it useful to promote these new systems within the hospital and serve as user liaisons on steering committees for information systems. Through this work, they could be able to transition into a new career in information systems.

The use of computers and information sciences by nurses worldwide is expanding quickly in the present day to help them carry out their ever-more-complex and sophisticated tasks. New roles for nurses are emerging in industry, research, system development, nursing education, nursing administration, and yes, even at the bedside, as a result of the development of nursing informatics. A common belief that information systems can be used to improve nursing practice and benefit patients by extending and improving the quality of care received is the driving force behind the entry of many nurses into the field of nursing informatics.

Definition

Hospital Information System are computer based software applications that integrate many medical, nursing, and administrative and miscellaneous functions of hospitals. It combines computer technology and communications to acquire and integrate financial and clinical data.

Nursing Information System are computer systems that manage clinical data from a variety of healthcare environments and made available in a timely and orderly fashion to aid nurses in improving patient care.

Purpose of Nursing Information Systems

- To make relevant patient data available in a usable form so patient care problems can be solved
- To process information to support management functions such as receiving data from departments and supplying data to departments to make policy decisions, operating decisions as well as patient care decisions
- To provide a comprehensive automated information processing system for all phases of the nursing process
- To develop care plan for families and patients

Components of Nursing Information Systems

- **Hardware:** Physical devices that provide handling function such as input, CPU, processing, storage or output of computer data.
- **Software:** Series of programming statements that perform a specific computer related application; categories include systems, operating, application and programming (word processors, spreadsheets, databases, multimedia applications and communication programs).
- **Network:** Devices and software applications that provide communication and data transfer between 2 or more computer systems. There are three types of networks:
- **Wide- Area Networks (WAN):** Are links to the outside world. They connect computer users to other users and systems through the telephone company's communication infrastructure. WAN support voice, data and image transmission.
- **Local- Area Network (LAN):** Are used to connect user's within

a local, somewhat defined, geographic area such as a building or closely grouped set of buildings.

• **Wireless networks connect information system:** Uses computer and communication hardware using wireless transmission of data, example electrocardiogram and cell phones

Examples of Nursing Information Systems

A System (EmSTAT) at Hennepin County Medical Center (Minnaeapolis, Minnesota) improves communication, facilitates continuity of care and decreases redundancy in documentation.

The Nursing Case Management Computerized System – an interactive computer program that enhances team planning of individualized care, decreased paperwork, aided the development of team care plans and facilitated improvements in the quality of patient care.

The Interactive Home Health Care systems- provide for audio and video interactions over local cable systems, as well as patient monitoring and data input and retrieval by the nurse.

NurseLink – an electronic bulletin board operated by the School of Nursing at the University of Colorado Health Sciences Center in Denver.

An Expert system – developed to assess pregnant women's risk of preterm birth.

Tips to develop Nursing Information Systems

• Choose software first

• Request software information from several vendors

• Provide vendor with pertinent information about size of agency, number of departments, type of departments and number of patients

• Provide information about the capabilities of the system users

- Provide information about other computerized systems within the organization
- Have the planning committee make a site visit to an organization where the selected software has been used
- Observe use of software in a similar organization
- Have vendor install, maintain and duplicate system information and train personnel
- Have vendor phase out former system

Nursing Information Systems Vs Emerging roles of nurses

Advances in information technology emphasized the need for all nurses to:

1. Incorporate data from evaluating patients' healthcare requirements

2. Creating care schedules

3. Giving other medical professionals access to patient data

4. Examining staffing and budget reports—nurses actually operate in an information-rich setting

5. Expanding one's understanding of health information concepts and the technology used to handle and process data

6. Nursing practice methods will adapt to take advantage of automation as technology continues to advance.

7. The frequent relocation of nursing professionals will play a crucial role in the integration of technology into the provision of patient care.

8. Because they collect and document data, have an understanding of global systems, set priorities, oversee all patient care, and recognize the importance of accessing patient information, nurses make excellent information systems personnel.

Issues related to Utilization of Nursing Information System

•Unfortunately, many of the earlier systems in use in hospitals and the marketplace have not satisfied the needs of nurses because, until recently, the nursing profession was not sufficiently involved in the selection, implementation, and decision-making regarding what systems are best for institutions.

• It is impossible to implement nursing informatics in a company without the employees experiencing the effects of the change.

• Despite the advantages nursing informatics offers, its use in healthcare is not common, and where it is, it has not been well received. This could be because end users are not properly informed about the rationale behind the technology's introduction and inadequate training is provided.

• There has been very little research done to evaluate the cost-effectiveness or cost-benefits of information systems.

• Problems with artificial intelligence and nursing informatics today are exacerbated by hypothetical future circumstances.

Strategies to Overcome the Issues

Five strategic directions recommended by the National Advisory Council on Nurse Education and Practice to enhance nurses' preparation to use and develop information technology:

1. To include care informatics content in nursing curriculum

2. To prepare nurses with specialized skills in informatics

3. To enhance nursing practice and education through informatics projects

4. To prepare nursing faculty in informatics

5. To increase collaborative efforts in nursing informatics

Nursing informatics, as a subset of health informatics in general, is a driving force behind the rapid changes that the nursing profession is experiencing. The nursing profession has further redefined competencies due to the expanded use of technology, creating opportunities for lifelong learning and requiring purpose-driven actions and a commitment-driven society. The automation of nursing data and information made possible by technology makes it possible to incorporate nursing information systems into every stage of patient care delivery. Nursing practice methods will adapt to take advantage of automation as technology advances. Nursing professionals will more frequently have key roles in integrating technology into patient care delivery. Not only will nurses be involved in the initial evaluation phases of information systems, but they will also play increasing roles in developing and sustaining the long term strategy for accessing patient information.

Evaluation and Analysis of Systematic Analysis of Healthcare

Big data has completely changed the way we live by opening up amazing possibilities for a wide range of uses. It contains an enormous amount of data, particularly a wide variety of data types that have been very helpful in many different research areas. Researchers in the healthcare field use computational tools to mine this data for enriched, pertinent information and create clever apps that quickly address pressing issues in the real world. The availability of new computational models and the availability of electronic health and mobile health facilities have made it possible for researchers and physicians to extract pertinent data and visualize healthcare big data in a new range of ways.

Researchers and caregivers face several challenges in the form of storage, minimizing treatment costs, and processing time (to extract enriched information, and minimize error rates to make optimum decisions) as a result of the digital transformation of healthcare systems through the use of information systems, medical technology, handheld, and smart wearable devices. This research project analyzes and evaluates the body of literature to find gaps that impair the overall effectiveness of the healthcare applications that are currently available. It also seeks to offer improved solutions to close these gaps. The current literature published between 2011 and 2021 is carefully examined in this extensive systematic research project to determine the efforts made to help medical professionals and doctors diagnose illnesses using big data analytics in healthcare.

In order to obtain successful results, a series of research questions are developed to analyze pertinent articles in order to pinpoint the salient characteristics and best practices for management. These analyses will then be applied later on. The systematic mapping's findings indicate that, in spite of the significant efforts made in the field of healthcare big data analytics, it is still necessary to adapt more recent hybrid machine learning-based systems and cloud computing-based models in order to lower treatment costs, shorten simulation times, and improve the quality of care. Additionally, by mapping data methodically, physicians, practitioners, researchers, and policymakers will be better equipped to use this study's findings as support for their own future research.

The burden of disease, overcrowding, and limited financial resources are putting tremendous strain on healthcare systems worldwide. The healthcare paradigm is changing in the current technological era from a traditional, one-size-fits-all approach to one that emphasizes personalized, individual care. Furthermore, there are variations in the quantity and nature of healthcare data. Healthcare providers handle lab results, imaging data, and other digital and analog data, such as ECG and MRI scans, in addition to the patient's medical history, physical examination, and other specific information.

This data is vast, comes in a variety of formats and types, and has a unique structure. These are the capabilities of Big Data to handle not only different types of and forms of data, but can handle 10 V structure including volume, variety, venue, varifocal, varmint, vocabulary, validity, volatility, veracity and velocity. Thus, the doctors facing an increasing burden of rising patient numbers coupled with progressively less time to spend with each patient. In other words, we are facing more patients, more data, and less time.

Big data has significantly impacted various fields, including healthcare, banking, and IoT, with an 80% increase in usage due to cloud sources, analytics, mobile technology, and social media technologies. Research on big data analytics in healthcare has shown potential in cognitive technology-based evaluations, brain hemorrhage detection, and accounting and business perspectives. Alharthi's review article explores Saudi Arabia's healthcare challenges and big data analytics applications, highlighting new applications and limited literature, primarily regional-specific. Systematic review process explores literature in various fields, but lacks significant work in healthcare big data domain to identify gaps and suggest future research directions.

The inspirational point that led us to pursue this systematic analysis was the pervasive and ubiquitous nature of big data. Efficient management and timely execution are the dire needs of big data, to extract enriched information regarding a certain problem of interest.

Many factors involved behind this systematic research work, but the most eminent reasons are:

1. The exiting research reported on big data does not provide significant information about the key features that should be considered to integrate both structured and unstructured big data in

healthcare domain. The pervasiveness of big data features challenging the researchers in pursuing research in this specialized domain. The underlying research on finding the key features will not only help in integrating big data in healthcare domain, but it will also assist in findings new gateways for future research directions.

2. Digital transformation of healthcare systems after the integration of information system, medical technology and other imaging systems have posed a big barrier for the research community in the form of a vast amount of information to deal with. While the over-population, limited data access, and disease burdens have restricted the doctors and practitioners to check more patients in a limited time. So, finding a suitable model that can efficiently process healthcare big data to extract information for a certain disease symptoms will not only helps the practitioners to suggest accurate medication and check more patients in timely manners, but it will open future research directions for the industrialists and policymakers to develop optimal healthcare big data processing models.

3. Accurate disease diagnosing by processing of gigantic amount of data, especially a plethora of types of data, within an interested processing domain is a key concern for both researchers and practitioners. Developing an efficient model that can accurately diagnose a certain by classifying images or other historical details of patients will not only helps the doctors to diagnose disease in timely manner and suggest medicine accordingly, but it will encourage the researchers and developers to develop an accurate disease identification model.

The remaining research paper is arranged as follows in the paper. The related work published in the suggested field is outlined in a section of the paper. The research framework used for this systematic investigation is presented in this section.

In the last few decades, information systems, medical technology, and other imaging resources have helped to bring about an unprecedented transformation of traditional healthcare systems into digital and portable healthcare applications. Big data are pushing healthcare organizations to adopt the extraction of pertinent information from other clinical records and imaginary data, which is drastically altering the healthcare system. With this data, accurate disease diagnosis will be produced at a high throughput, treatment costs will drop, and availability will rise.

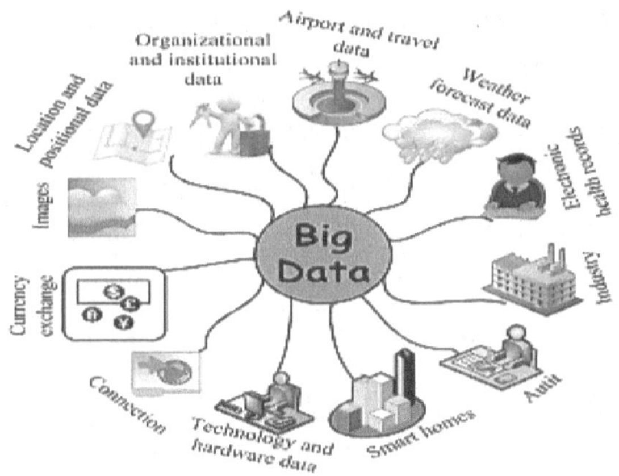

Figure- Main steps of the research protocol.

When the term "big data" was first used in the context of data visualization in 1997, it presented legislators and medical professionals with an extraordinary and ambitious task, with a focus on personalized medicine. However, data collection is happening more quickly than data analysis or processing, highlighting the growing disparity between the quick advancement of technology in data collection and the relatively slow functional characterization of medical records. In this sense, the historical data from an individual patient's electronic health records (EHR), including phonotypical and other genomic data, is becoming increasingly important. The main sources of large data are shown in the figure.

This systematic analysis is performed using the following preliminary steps:

•   Identification of research questions to systematically analyze the proposed field from different perspectives.

•   Selection of relevant keywords and queries to download the most relevant research articles.

•   Selection of peer-reviewed online databases to download relevant research articles published in healthcare big data domain during the period ranging from 2011 – 2021.

•   Perform inclusion and exclusion process based on title, abstract and the contents presented in the article to remove duplicate records.

•   Assess the finalized relevant articles for identifying gaps in the available literature and suggest new research directions to explore.

A few researchers begin downloading articles and defend a general query (32, 33). Even though gathering articles from internet databases is straightforward, most of the most pertinent articles are frequently missed. Therefore, defining keywords for every research question is the right course of action. Although it is a demanding job, the end result is the retrieval of every pertinent article related to a particular research problem from online databases.

Formulation of Search String

Search strings (queries) are formulated using the keywords identifed from the selected research questions. Te search string is tested in online databases and was modifed according to retrieve each relevant articles from these databases. Inspired from the guidelines proposed by Wohlin33, following are the key steps undertaken to develop an optimal search string: i. Identifcation of key terms from the formulated topic and research questions ii. Selection of alternate words or synonyms for key terms iii. Use "OR" operator for alternating words or synonyms during query formation iv. Link all major terms with Boolean "AND" operator to validate every single keyword. Following all these preliminary steps a generic query/search-string is developed that is depicted in Table 2.

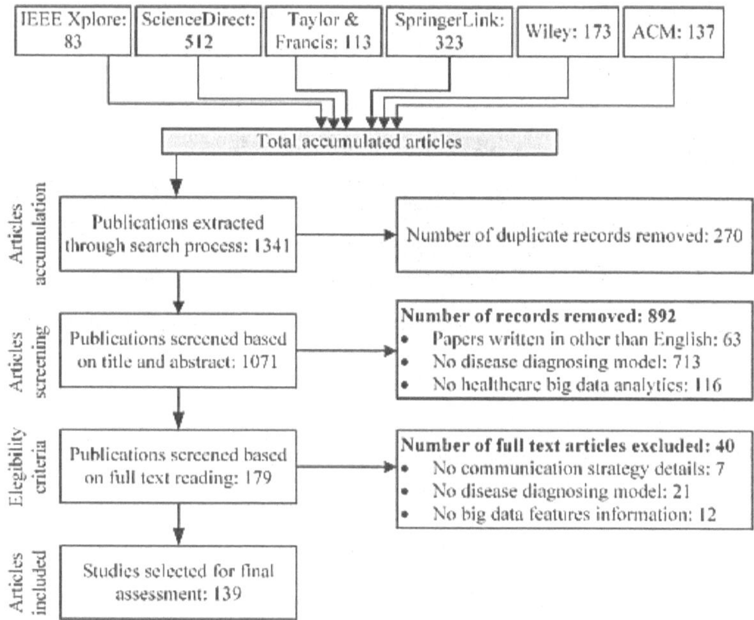

Figure- PRISMA process model for articles accumulation, screening, and fnal selection

Tis generic query is further refned for each research question as depicted in Table 3 to retrieve each relevant article. Selection of online repositories. Afer identifying keywords and formulating search strings the next step is to download relevant articles specifc to the interested research problem. For the accumulation of relevant articles six well-known and peer-reviewed online repositories are selected, as depicted in Table 3. Articles accumulation and fnal database development. For relevant articles accumulation and fnal database development we followed the guidelines suggested by Kable et al.34. Afer specifying the research questions, identifying keywords, and formulating search queries, and selecting online repositories, the next key step is to develop a relevant articles database for the analysis and assessment purposes that includes three prime steps:

(1) identifcation of inclusion/exclusion criteria for a certain research article(s), and

(2) Relevant articles database development.

Below is a detailed discussion of these steps. criteria for inclusion and exclusion. Once the author(s) has chosen an online database and initiated the process of downloading articles, the most arduous task they must undertake is determining which particular paper should be included in the final database or not. In order to address this issue, inclusion and exclusion criteria are defined for each article before it can be included in the final collection of articles. The writers use a manual procedure to decide which articles should be included and which should be excluded. These articles are assessed according to the information presented in the abstract, title, and body of the paper. If more than half authors agree upon the inclusion of a certain article based on these parameters (title, abstract, and contents presented in the article), then that paper was counted in the fnal database otherwise rejected. A total of 134 relevant primary studies are selected for the fnal assessment process. To ensure no skip of relevant article snowballing is applied to retrieve each relevant article

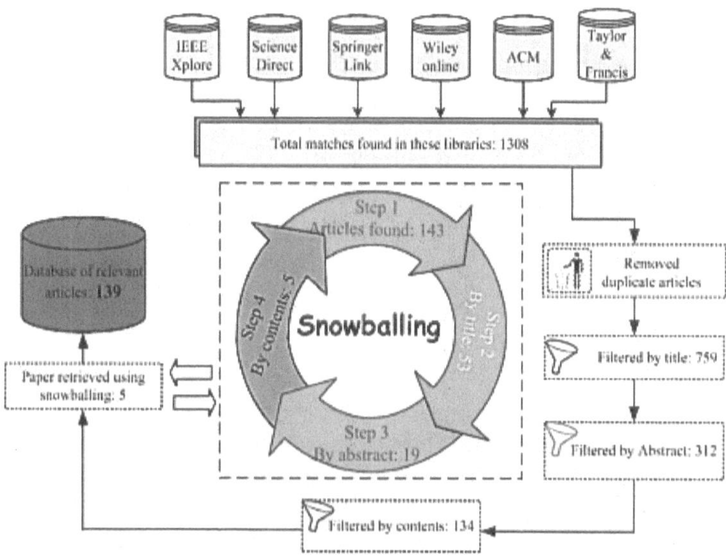

Fig- presentations of snowballing

Limitations Tis article has a number of limitations. Some of these limitations are listed below.

• For this systematic analysis articles are only accumulated from six diferent peer-reviewed libraries (ACM, SpringerLink, Taylor & Francis, Science Direct=IEEE Xplore, and Wiley online library), but there exist a number of multi-disciplinary databases for articles accumulation purposes.

• Tis systematic analysis covers a specifc range of years (2011 – 2021), while a number of articles are reporting on daily basis.

• Articles are accumulated from online libraries using search queries, so if a paper has no matching words to the query, then it was skipped during search process.

• Google Scholar is skipped during the articles accumulation phase to shorten the searching time. Also, it gives access to both peer-reviewed and non-peer-reviewed journals and we only focused on peer-reviewed journals for the relevant articles.

• Being a systematic literature work it can be broadened to grab the knowledge about other varying topics such as healthcare data commercialization, health sociology etc.

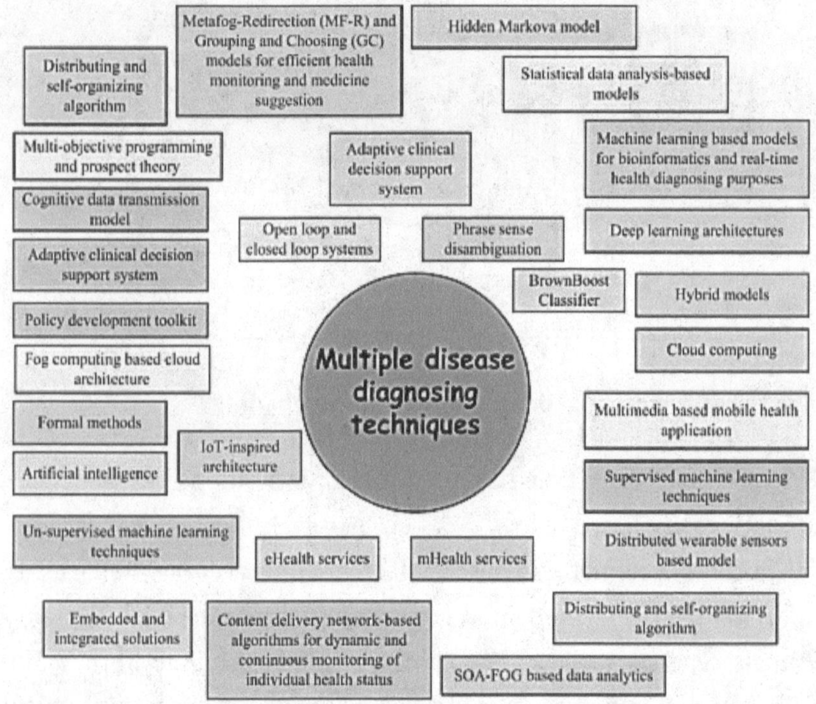

Figure- Multiple disease diagnosing techniques proposed in the literature.

Final thoughts and upcoming projects This research article provides a thorough analysis of the published research from 2011 to 2021, highlighting the efforts made by scientists to support physicians and caregivers in making accurate diagnoses of diseases and recommending appropriate medications. The researchers proposed multiple frameworks for feature extraction, identification, and remote communication based on the research problem and underlying requirements to facilitate timely development of doctor-patient communication. Big data analytics and computing devices are the main tools used in these real-time or almost real-time applications. In order to achieve successful outcomes in the diagnosis of disease, this research work identified a number of critical features and optimal management designs suggested in the healthcare big data analytical domain. The findings of this methodical study indicate that in order to lower treatment costs, shorten simulation times, and enhance care quality, sophisticated hybrid machine learning-based models and cloud computing applications should be modified. The results of this study will support the development of sophisticated disease diagnosis models by researchers and practitioners, as well as the presentation of better treatment options to patients by policymakers. High-tech hybrid machine learning frameworks for cognitive computing are thought to be the next generation of tools for data-driven big data analysis in healthcare. Additionally, geometric features rather than semantic and structural features should be taken into account when extracting features. These geometric-based feature extraction techniques will shorten the simulation time while simultaneously enhancing the smart health devices' capacity for identification and illness diagnosis. Furthermore, these characteristics can be used in conjunction with advanced machine learning and big data analytics to accurately identify Alzheimer's disease and tumors in PET or MRI images. For data organization purposes, cluster-based mechanisms should be taken into consideration to enhance big data's management and timely access capabilities. Future innovation in the healthcare sector will depend heavily on the promotion of research in these areas.

Chapter-9

Information Law & Governance in Clinical Practice

Ethical- Legal Issues Pertaining to Health Care Information in Clinical Practice

Due to the fact that patient safety is multifaceted and based on moral and legal requirements, it is important to consider both moral and legal issues. Experts from a variety of fields discussed the ethical and legal aspects of patient safety after a 12-day-old newborn's falling incident case came up during the monthly ethics round at Tehran University of Medical Sciences, Iran's Children's Medical Center.

This report discusses various facets of patient safety, including risk management and root cause analysis (RCA), the importance of professionalism and human resources, the need to notify parents of medical errors, and forensic medicine with an emphasis on ethical issues.

The non-maleficence principle of medical ethics states that a healthcare provider's top priority should be protecting their patients from harm and preventing injury. As a result, it has received the greatest attention as a factor in the global quality of healthcare services. After the Institute of Medicine (IOM) published a report in 1999 titled "Man is fallible: create a safe health system" regarding the prevalence of medical errors in the United States, patient safety became a global movement. In response, the Iranian health care system put in place unique plans with the goal of providing standard medical services, avoiding errors, and organizing a methodical approach to risk management, systematic deficiency, and patient safety improvement. One of these programs is clinical governance which was introduced by the Ministry of Health and Medical Education (MOHME) and initiated since November 2009. Although great emphasis has been placed on the importance of clinical governance by the MOHME, there are some challenges in achieving the desired outcomes. This could be the result of healthcare providers' inadequate understanding about the importance of clinical governance and lack of organizational safety culture.

Research findings indicate that a significant proportion of patients experience injuries related to medical care. A World Health Organization (WHO) report states that there is a 1 in 300 chance of injuring patients while providing medical care, compared to a 1 in 100,000 chance of aviation accidents. Since the patient safety project started in 2004, more than 140 nations have made an effort to enhance the safety plans for their own healthcare systems. Errors with medications and falls are the most common causes of injuries. Just 4% of incidents are considered serious, despite falling accounting for 21% of all incidents. Meanwhile the neonatal falling statistics in the USA is 1.6-4.4 in 10,000 live births, an estimated 600-1600 falling incidents in a year. These cases are often the result of shortcomings in systems and processes, organizational complexity and ambiguity, and poor communication.

The ethical and legal implications of this matter receive less attention despite the numerous patient safety guidelines and standards that exist. The primary objective of patient safety in the healthcare system can be examined from two angles from a moral standpoint. It can be examined as a practical value since its advantages and good effects are the primary concern. By concentrating on the defense and advancement of humanity and human dignity, it can also be examined as a moral principle. It is imperative to underscore the significance of both facets within the healthcare system. From a professional perspective, moral principles pertaining to patient safety are not distinct from fundamental medical duties; in fact, they are so fundamental that they may serve as the foundation for other moral principles that are stressed in medicine. This indicates that the idea of human dignity and patient safety are strongly related, and that any precautions taken for patient safety must also ensure that human dignity is protected. Stated differently, there exists a close relationship between human dignity and the professional commitment and responsibility of healthcare personnel.

Experts from a variety of fields discussed the ethical aspects of patient safety when this case was brought up during the monthly ethics round at Tehran University of Medical Sciences in Tehran, Iran. The viewpoints presented in this article are a compilation of the opinions of specialists in a number of disciplines, including nursing, medical law, neonatology, and ethics. It is noteworthy to mention that the Children's Medical Center has been holding its monthly ethics round for over five years. Every session includes a discussion of a complex case involving a variety of pertinent experts.

The clinical case

Multiple seizures led to the hospitalization of a 12-day-old newborn infant in the neonatal intensive care unit (NICU). He was the family's firstborn child. There was no history of seizures or any other illness in the mother's or family's past. Medication was used to control the seizures, and electroencephalography (EEG) and other diagnostic tests were ordered. The baby was supposed to be moved to the level II NICU since he was stable and had tolerated breast feeding, but this was delayed because there weren't enough beds available.

His nurse discovered the infant was on the floor and the incubator door was open when she heard a loud noise during the third day of admission's evening shift. The incident was promptly reported to the on-call physician by the charge nurse. After a thorough examination, no physical injuries were discovered on the newborn. Additionally, the incident was reported to the department's chief physician, and hospital administrators received a copy of the incident report right away. Later, to ensure they were sufficiently secure, all other incubators were examined. The mother had claimed that she was sleeping when the incident occurred, but when the staff told the newborn's father about the fall, he accused the mother of abandoning the child.

Root Cause Analysis and Risk Management

One of the first and most important steps taken to reduce the frequency of patient injuries is looking for the causes and coming up with the best solution, or, to put it another way, doing a basic analysis of the incident. It should be highlighted that the aforementioned procedure needs to be impartial and concentrate on determining the root cause and finding a solution rather than assigning blame. Having specific guidelines for reporting the incident in a proper, organized, ethical setting without making accusations against anyone is one way to stop such incidents. Indeed, there are a number of obstacles that prevent hospital staff members from reporting medical errors, including guilt feelings, sanctions, a lack of organizational support, poor feedback, and ignorance of the contributing variables.

Numerous factors affect the evaluation and mitigation of patients' risk of harm, also known as risk management in the clinical setting. Creating an organizational culture in all hospital levels that is predicated on effective communication and mutual trust is one approach. From an ethical standpoint, effective risk management requires the value of reliability. Given that it relates to cultural, psychological, and physical safety, this value is associated with safety culture. Therefore, in order to enhance patient safety and care quality, managers have an obligation to establish open and honest mental and physical safety environments. In order to promote transparent reporting, managers should also strongly encourage interdisciplinary collaboration.

Developing policies and procedures that are tailored to the specific needs of each ward is the most crucial step in lowering the likelihood of such incidents in clinical settings. Other actions that can be taken in this regard include steady supervision, ongoing training of staff members in patient safety, and monitoring the degree of efficacy of actions performed. For example, in this situation, it's crucial to regularly check the incubator door, use two locks, and give staff members instructions on incubator safety. Additionally, feedback and ongoing monitoring of adherence to patient safety regulations are required.

The role of human resources

The quantity of human resources is also noteworthy in the field of patient safety. In other words, quality assurance depends on the quantity of manpower. Therefore, in order to prevent similar incidents, providing an adequate number of staff at the bedside is essential .

The role of professionalism

Fundamental ideas in medicine are intertwined with professional ethics and patient safety. Patient safety is based on moral standards, which are markers of high-quality healthcare. A professional code of ethics must be established and followed in order to achieve patient safety. The Iranian healthcare professional code of conduct stipulates that every patient must receive dignified treatment and be shielded from any potential harm. Therefore, in order to prevent falling incidents, healthcare providers must identify potential safety failures in accordance with ethical principles. There are various organizational, professional, and individual components to establishing patient safety, with an emphasis on ethics. A commitment to professionalism and organization facilitates the recognition and reporting of mistakes made by oneself and by others.

From an ethical view, the following actions are recommended:

Observing any professional or institutional guidelines pertaining to incidents involving falls; executing fundamental measures to evaluate the patient's physical condition and preserve his or her life; notifying the staff member in charge; The situation should be assessed promptly, and all relevant information should be recorded and reported, including the time of the incident, the infant's position, consciousness level, vital signs, the people who were present, the steps taken during the process, and so forth; Notifying the parents and offering them emotional assistance.

Informing parents (Disclosure of medical errors)

It appears that if the care team makes a mistake, it needs to be openly disclosed to the parents, without placing the blame on the caregivers. Furthermore, it is best to avoid using grating expressions like "It happens" and "Nothing has happened though." In cases where mistakes were brought about by an improper pattern of hospital service delivery, parents should be assured that the hospital will cover the full cost of all services. It would be preferable if the head nurse or chief physician told the parents and gave them ample opportunity to voice their worries or frustrations.

Although anger under such circumstances is a natural reaction, we cannot hide medical errors because of fear of parents' reaction. Moreover, parents' anger would be more severe if they found out that the hospital personnel have concealed the truth.

It should be recognized that one of the fundamental rights of patients and their families is to know the truth. Similar studies suggest that informing patients about the error may cause a stressful scenario along with strong emotional responses from the patient, family, or the healthcare team. In most cases, the patient or family members feel angry and anxious, and the person who made the mistake feels guilty or afraid of punishment. Furthermore, it should be noticed that primary conversations usually take place when there is not accurate and comprehensive information about the event, so recognizing, understanding, and explaining all the details in complicated clinical situations is not possible. Thus, it is suggested that in such situations, information be given in several stages and by providing psychological support for the patient.

Moreover, the patient's family can be regarded as a valuable source of information in the process of root cause analysis (RCA) of comparable incidents, even though they might require supportive interventions. Actively collaborating with the patient's family may be a high-yield strategy for identifying and preventing medical errors, as ensuring ethical patient safety is a multifaceted task.

In addition, regarding the presented case, the father should be ensured that hospitalizing the newborn was necessary and the mother should not be blamed. In fact, he should be ensured that the incident was entirely due to system error and not by the mother. Basically, maintaining the integrity of the family is essential and medical staff must consider family support at all stages, especially in such circumstances.

The need to apologize honestly is, in fact, a crucial ethical consideration in this situation. Saying "We are sorry" is not always enough. Healthcare professionals urgently need to be trained in sensitive interpersonal relationships and related skills in order to facilitate appropriate and honest communication with the patient's family, as informing the parents is a delicate matter.

Forensic medicine aspect

Patient safety laws and regulations, which differ depending on the legal framework of each nation, ought to promote the reporting of medical errors and aid in the application of the moral requirements of patient safety. Medical law generally stipulates that a patient who suffers harm as a result of negligence should receive just compensation. Furthermore, these regulations offer avenues for encouraging openness and transparency in communication at all levels. All parties involved in the healthcare system must be considered in order to achieve this goal.

In the mentioned case, some questions could be raised. Either the falling was in the presence of the mother or not. If it was in her presence, the hypothesis is that she dropped the baby intentionally. However, if there is no sign of any apparent trauma, it seems there was no specific hurtful force or he fell from his mother's arms, and it shows the mother's lack of experience.

Therefore, it should be acknowledged that one of the main risk factors for newborn falls is postpartum sleepiness in mothers. In half of all newborn falls that happen in hospitals, the mother was holding the baby while it was in bed. As a result, one of the main duties of nurses is to identify the risks of neonatal falls during mother-baby care situations and to educate the mothers. Should the mother be unable to care for her hospitalized child, the care team should supervise her and provide her with education. Furthermore, if the father brought up the complaint, it is appropriate to notify him.

Following a thorough examination and treatment, the doctor's or nurse's primary responsibility is to meticulously record and describe every incident without making any assumptions. It would be a whole different conversation and would be imperative to contact social services if the examinations revealed evidence of neglect.

In a healthcare setting, it is required to notify the patient or their family of any unwelcome event. The conventional view of the law supports the notion that errors that did not impact the patient do not need to be disclosed. Furthermore, it is now widely recognized that making these kinds of disclosures will increase patients' trust in medical professionals while also educating them about the world around them. Additionally, by using this strategy, medical staff members can respect the autonomy and dignity of their patients.

There are still many risks to patient safety in healthcare settings, even with the focus on the quality of care services receiving more attention. Due to the fact that patient safety is multifaceted and based on moral and legal requirements, it is important to consider both moral and legal issues.

It takes structured policies and procedures to promote the safety settings based on mutual trust in order to achieve the healthcare system's ultimate goal, which is to ensure the quality and safety of the services. Promoting interdisciplinary cooperation for the open reporting of medical errors as well as the active involvement of patients and their families in the identification of medical errors can help with this. Furthermore, the provision of emotional support and legal protection of the staffs by the organization is essential to encourage voluntary reporting of incidents.

Legal and Ethical Issues in Health Informatics

Federal, state, and local laws, in addition to an ethical code disseminated by the American Health Information Management Association (AHIMA), serve as guidelines for health informatics practitioners.

Keeping up with legal and ethical issues can be difficult in this relatively new profession that is changing quickly due to rapid technological advancements. Among the professional communities impacted by changing rules, laws, and ethical standards are medical researchers, health policymakers, and healthcare professionals and consultants.

The American Medical Informatics Association (AMIA) places a lot of emphasis on these topics and provides its members with a working group dedicated to continuing education regarding ethical, legal, and social issues pertaining to health informatics.

Every aspect of the health informatics profession is affected in some way by ethical and legal concerns. The issue essentially comes down to finding a way to balance the need to protect the security of patient information with the potential for better care and outcomes associated with greater **interoperability** and improved ability to share records among healthcare entities.

The foundation of the health informatics field is the belief that patients and healthcare professionals shouldn't have to choose between record security and sharing convenience. This is a high-level view of the overall objective of health informatics specialists, whose main duty is to support the healthcare sector in integrating electronic medical records in a safe and effective manner.

Over the past ten years, as the profession has become more well-known, rules and standards for ethical behavior have been updated and expanded. Because of this, graduates of today's health informatics programs have an extensive array of specialization options at their disposal.

Here are a just a few of the ethical, legal and social issues that are shaping the **health informatics profession** today:

- The protection of private patient information
- Patient safety
- Risk assessment
- Reporting design and data display
- System implementation
- Curriculum development
- Research ethics
- Liability
- User involvement and accessibility
- Ethical dilemmas resulting from data availability and sharing

Existing health informatics-related laws

The Privacy Act of 1974 is among the most significant laws in effect today that have an impact on health informatics. According to this law, federal agencies must publish notice of their records systems in the Federal Register to give the public notice of them. Additionally, it stipulates a procedure for subjects to access or modify their records and demands their written consent before a record can be released.

Other important regulatory rulings and organizations include:

• The Confidentiality of Alcohol and Drug Abuse Patient Records regulations, which provided additional protections of privacy for patients in substance abuse treatment programs regulated by the federal government

• The Institutional Review Board (IRB), which are established by various government health sciences bodies (federal and/or state) to protect rights, welfare and well-being of human research participants and patients

• The Joint Commission on Accreditation of Healthcare Organizations (the Joint Commission), which rules on the eligibility of hospitals and other organizations to participate in Medicare

• The Health Information Technology for Economic and Clinical Health (HITECH) Act, which was enacted in 2009 as part of the American Recovery and Reinvestment Act to promote the adoption of health information technology, as well as to ensure compliance on the institutional level

• The Health Insurance Portability and Accountability Act (HIPAA), which strengthened the privacy protections of patients regarding the sharing of medical information, particularly as it relates to employment

• The Food and Drug Administration Safety and Innovation Act (FDASIA), which in 2012 strengthened the FDA's ability to speed patient access to digital records and improve the safety of drugs, medical devices, and biological products

• The 21st Century Cures Act, which became law in December 2016 and is designed to accelerate the development of medical technology and improve patient access to technological advances in medicine

Laws and regulations are closely tied to ethical concerns. Several health information technology organizations – AHIMA, AMIA and the Health Information Management and Systems Society (HIMSS) — have taken on leadership roles for the examination and implementation of ethical standards in the industry.

The Code of Ethics and Standards

According to the Code of Ethics, a health information management (HIM) professional's ethical duties include protecting the confidentiality and security of patient data, disclosing patient data, developing, utilizing, and maintaining patient data systems, and guaranteeing the accuracy and accessibility of patient data.

It also gives seven purposes for the code of ethics:

• The promotion of high standards of health information management practice

• The identification of core values of the health information management mission

• A summary of the broad ethical principles that reflect the core values

• Establishment of ethical principles used to guide decisions and actions

• Establishment of a framework for professional resolution of conflicts and ethical uncertainties

• Providing ethical principles that allow the public to hold health information management professionals accountable

• Providing opportunities for mentors to guide new practitioners in ethics education

Legal matters

In 2013, Nancy J. Brent—a writer, columnist, lawyer, and nurse—published a list of crucial legal considerations for health informatics professionals on the HIMSS website. Brent's guidance was distilled into these key points:

• The highest priority for a health information management team must be patient safety.

• Procedures for health information management must be established, and team members must be well-trained on these policies.

- Patient information much be held as securely as possible.
- Passwords and other login information must never be shared among team members.

Brent also suggests that health informatics professionals stay up to date on new laws and decisions pertaining to ethical disputes and uncertainties in the industry. Front-line health informatics professionals' depth of knowledge is critical to protecting patient rights and advancing the use of electronic technology to improve health outcomes.

Healthcare professionals can help shape the future of health information management with a Master of Science in Health Informatics from USF Health Morsani College of Medicine, offered 100% online. Trained professionals are becoming more and more necessary for healthcare organizations to design and implement records systems that safeguard patient privacy and facilitate data sharing among stakeholders.

Chapter-10

Health Quality & Evidence Based Practice

Improving the Quality of Healthcare by Using Information Technology System in Health Care

The rapid advancement of information technology, coupled with the invasion of the world during the so-called globalization era, has given rise to terminology that has evolved to describe how people use digital technologies and computer devices for their own benefit and to improve the way they live their lives. This helps IT enhance service delivery procedures, facilitating and facilitating the work and transactions that hospitals provide to its auditors and achieving communication with them. This allows for the transparent and clear provision of data and information to the auditors, as well as the provision of models and procedures to improve service delivery, which eases the process of dealing with employees.

Everybody knows that the IT system is crucial to every aspect of our everyday lives and activities. Because of the influence the IT system has on the health care industry, it has been used as an example. Later on in this study, we shall observe. Our information technology system is still quite basic in comparison to many developed countries, despite the fact that they use IT systems in the same industry. One of the world's most significant ecosystems is the IT system. Because of advances in the use of information technology in recent years and the increasing sophistication in all areas of life, this service has made it possible for many people to communicate directly with one another and search in global libraries, scientific journals, websites, and other important features, the basic benefit of this system is to improve the quality of health care.

The nature of the relationship between independent and dependent variables is demonstrated by this study. A perfect positive correlation or perfect negative correlation between two variables was found by running a person correlation between the variables to ascertain the relationship between them. The researcher carried out this investigation to determine whether or not any correlation between two variables is significant, even though it may range between -1.0 and +1.0. Because health services have a direct impact on people's health, it is imperative that they be provided at a higher standard and at a lower cost to all due to the growing population. The "efficiency of health workers" is one example of these techniques used to improve health care.

Improving the standard of care and patients' satisfaction with this service rank among the top priorities for the health care industry. Other concerns, like performance efficiency gained from this service's availability and its facilitation in the healthcare industry, could enhance this field's IT system. "We have observed a fast and growing evolution of the IT system in all sectors in the past few years, which makes the provision of health services challenging."

The researcher observed that staff members are not using the IT system to its full potential both at the outset of the study and following the completion of a survey among workers at Yemeni hospitals located in the country's capital, Sana'a. The investigator came to the conclusion that there may not have been many prior studies in this area. In this study, we observe the function of the IT system and its direct influence on the healthcare industry. The emergence of the aforementioned issue has made it necessary to look for technological tools that, when applied as demonstrated in the literature, could aid in improving Yemeni hospitals' IT systems.

In order to encourage hospitals to utilize information technology in the right ways, it is also necessary to look for scientific proof by assessing the system's tools and its effects on healthcare. From the perspective of the researcher, the study's knowledge gap is that the capital Sanaa hospitals' use of information technology systems has an effect on the caliber of care they provide.

"Health care is one of the most important challenges and difficulties facing most of the world, especially developing countries," states the statement. "The public sector contains many basic and important elements, of which health care is the most important component." Working across institutional, professional, and geographic barriers to effectively collaborate and coordinate is one of the biggest challenges facing the health care industry these days. Numerous advantages can be realized, and certain aspects of health care are universally addressed, such as better patient access to care and higher-quality prescription drugs.

Healthcare System

Healthcare systems are institutions that provide medical treatments, such as equipment and residential care, along with additional services to treat patients. These days, there are so many options available for health care systems that making a decision can frequently be quite challenging. The World Health Organization (WHO) defines the health system as "a system comprising all entities, individuals, and initiatives whose main goal is to maintain, restore, or advance health."

A rapid and significant change was observed in the health care sector where the situation became worse and chronic health problems worsened over time. The medical system is a specialized system that includes a number of specialized personnel in different fields, through which they facilitate medical services and provide the necessary health care. It is not without complications that accompany this system.

The health care system is one of the most complex systems, Health care systems are considered one of the most complex systems through coordination between the hospital and outside hospitals, which work hard to provide the appropriate service to the patient.

The most reliant system in this industry is now the health care systems in many of the world's recent introductions of IT. The health sector has a significant adoption rate of the information technology system, which is used exceptionally well in the medical field. These days, a lot of hospitals use IT systems that support and ease the work of medical personnel.

Despite global challenges, health care providers offer support in the field of information technology on health systems. Worldwide adoption of the Internet and other information technologies, including electronic registration systems, is essential to the functioning of the healthcare system. Many developed nations have made significant financial investments to support the adoption of electronic health care systems.

The Reasons for the Increased Adoption of the IT System in the Health Sector

A major change in the health sector is the use of information technology systems, which are predicted to become the most popular in the coming years. These systems will offer a host of facilities and, most importantly, allow patients to take an active role in their care. According to researcher Viitanen, being comfortable with the health technology system will help to improve the quality of care given by easing the burden on staff members and facilitating their roles. However, we should know that there are several factors that directly effect on the adoption of the IT system in the field of health care. The researcher found the following factors:-The first factor, As a result of the rapid development of information technology, this has led to the adoption of technology in most sectors of government and the most important sectors of health and this may cause a significant change in the quality of health care. The second factor is to reduce the budget of certain equipment used as sensors and screens.

The third is the quick and efficient sharing of health information via telecommunications systems, which is made possible by the increasing and rapid use of Internet networks and network information systems. The fourth factor is that patients will receive direct care, particularly for personal health needs. The fifth factor makes it possible to access all information systems and use wireless communication devices.

It also presents fantastic chances to obtain insightful feedback that can be used to raise patient satisfaction and healthcare quality. In order to improve self-patient management there are new opportunities for the patient to receive appropriate advice via the use of feedback. The sixth factor, recently, the information technology system in the health care sector has become a target for all users for all purposes because it contains a wide range of services and applications .

Seven factors, as the use of the computer system in all sectors of the state increases, the IT system can occupy an important place in health care sectors. Finally, many benefits may be obtained from ICT in healthcare, as we will see later in this research.

Challenges Facing Healthcare area with Adoption and Usage of ICT

Dealing with all the various fields and concentrating on the use of information technology in healthcare can present a number of challenges. The researcher will briefly summarize his findings from several earlier works of literature.

Numerous nations worldwide are attempting to implement technology in the healthcare industry, but there are numerous obstacles that need to be overcome before doing so. Thus, the implementation appears to be very challenging.

Some of the challenges that appear when using a video connection technique to be:

1) The difficulty of direct contact.

2) Lack of knowledge of the technology leading to the reluctance to use self-care.

3) The quality of video usage is unclear due to a poor internet connection.

4) Lack of some skills such as motor skills and knowledge.

Returning to Viitanen , the difficulties faced by the public whether developed or developing when using the IT system in the health care sector are as follows:

1) Demonstration of complex medical data.

2) Some problems in the process of inserting and outputting data.

3) Security Complexities.

4) There is no clear identity for the patient.

5) Insufficient awareness of the benefits and risk of this technical information.

Omary found out that some of the challenges faced by developed and developing countries using the IT system in the health care sector are as follows:

1) lack of clear identity for the patient.

2) Poverty and lack of Internet availability, which is significant.

3) Lack of health care policy in the medical sectors.

4) Lacks international standards.

5) The existence of security complications.

The primary issue with the application of IT systems in developing nations was their lack of funding, despite the fact that these systems' implementation is straightforward and doable in developing nations; however, due to the unique conditions and factors of developed nations, where the majority of tests and implementation originate, implementation becomes problematic.

Impact of Information Technology System on Health Care

• Information Technology in General

The advancement of science and industry continues to progress at a rapid pace, with one of the most significant recent developments being the resurgence of IT system use. Research demonstrates that "the health care sector has experienced problems due to the rapid progress in the IT system." The researcher points out that utilizing IT systems in our daily lives has a number of advantages.

The information technology system in the health sector is being used increasingly. It has great importance in improving the quality of care and in caring for patients. Information work is the main and important item in the health care sector, Hence we note its importance as a dense industry for the use of information. When a patient visits a health care center, it is based on a digital or paper version containing health information about the patient (patient health information PHI). This is considered one of the most important difficulties facing the general medical staff and the private doctor in wasting time by collecting data. In addition to this, the nurse should play a large role by providing consultation or cooperation with doctors in all specialties. In case of need of doctors or nurses for some health, information should be available at anytime and anywhere and clearly.

From this point on, HIS can be described as a specialized task management system used in the healthcare industry. The implementation of an IT system has affected clinical work in hospitals. It is crucial for the Department of Patient Care Management's computerized system and data collection.

An electronic system with a variety of uses and functions is one of the most significant systems that depends on documents and papers (HIS). It might include a number of subsystems, like a laboratory information system, in addition to one or more specialized computer applications. One of the most crucial elements in this field is the clear coordination of the data. The health system calendar is dependent on accurate information systems and pertinent health data, which demonstrates how well it improves quality and reduces medical errors. It also plays a part in resource distribution by facilitating genuine coordination.

Information Technology Background

The last few days have seen a rise in the use of contemporary communication tools like smartphones and the Internet. In order to facilitate information sharing across the health and other sectors, infrastructure for information technology is crucial. Thus, we observe that wealthy nations are interested in seeing the growth and investment of telecommunications infrastructure in all systems, particularly the health care delivery system. All health sector staff, whether administrative or clinical, must diversify the collection of patient information and adopt different sources for this purpose. Communication must be maintained between all hospital departments and all related departments. Health care services are widely distributed, but there is a notable presence for many specialists in all specialties, this indicates the importance of sharing and sharing information among health and patient workers.

The working personnel cooperate and work together to take advantage of the network's characteristics in the health sector. The integration of information technology, network communications, and healthcare facilities is one of the most crucial strategies to enhance healthcare. There is also an important way to improve the health of citizens and manage their patients through continuous interaction between service providers and patients.

The provision of health care services depends on the cooperation of the shareholders in this service through organizational boundaries. Also, "Through experience and studies proved that patients who consult a health sector resort to treatment and stay in another health hospital for different reasons". Until a proper diagnosis is obtained and given effective medication there is a need for coordination and good communication between work activities in all health care sectors.

The significance of processes for coordination, whether done directly or via an electronic system It facilitates processing and conservation as well as diagnosis and data access, allowing service recipients to participate in the process. According to Nicola and Jarke, the distributed information system is a valuable tool for determining a patient's overall health and making general disease diagnoses.

Tools are Using in Healthcare

Many tools are used in the health care sector and this may be done directly or indirectly, as many depend on them, such as using the Internet, for example using the e-mail tool.

In addition, there are direct ways to benefit from this care by means of direct communication such as mobile phone use. We can point out that no matter how different the tools are but give the same effect, in this part we will discuss the tools that affect the use of the IT system in the sector Health care and focus on the importance of these tools and we can summarize as follows:

Internet, Electronic Mail (E-Mail), Health Web Portals, Electronic Health Records (EHR). Telemedicine or Telehealth, Mobile Health (M-health), and Mobile Phone.

• Internet

Technology, particularly computers and the Internet, will play a major role in the health sector in the future. The idea of management has evolved in a contemporary way as a result of the Internet, technology, and the recent period of rapid development. The Internet has grown in significance for both patients and doctors due to its ability to provide information retrieval at any time.

The Internet has become a valuable resource for the health care industry due to its constant and widespread use, as well as its growing utilization in all fields. This has made it possible to access the medical information that is required. Where everyone now has access to information in all fields, particularly in the medical field. There are many websites that may reach 100,000 sites worldwide and each site contains a variety of health information that may benefit consumers or beneficiaries There are also many Internet users around the world using the Internet to search and choose the best and most appropriate health information .

We note that due to the rapid development of technology usage many service providers rely heavily on the use of the Internet.

• Electronic Mail (E-Mail)

One of the most useful tools is email, which serves a variety of purposes and is appropriate in many situations, including non-emergency situations, since it allows users to store electronic records and data and retrieve them as needed. The use of email in the medical field has increased noticeably recently, and it helps to improve communication between doctors who practice in different specialties or the same one, as well as between patients and physicians. It serves the two primary functions of scheduling appointments and delivering test results. It serves the two primary functions of scheduling appointments and delivering test results.

One of the important things that may facilitate the patient who has the ability to use the Internet is to inquire about any examination or any health problem with email and receive the answer from the doctor. Here we note that the provision of email has special importance in engaging patients in the health care sector.

The usage of email services helped to solve this issue because doctors frequently do not have enough time to spend with their patients. As a result, a lot of patients use email to take notice of a doctor's important consultation. The information obtained from the doctor via the website is more advantageous than that obtained through other channels because it may provide a detailed explanation of the case, which the patient can retain and use as a reference when needed.

• Health Web Portals

One of the busiest pages on websites are active server pages (ASPs), which are frequented by many users who use them to find the answers. They can evaluate the patient's data using this program and advise him to see a physician.Due to its ease of use for both audio and video communication, it is regarded as one of the most significant forms of electronic communication.

The use of healthy web portals is one of the most crucial e-health adoption strategies that raises the standard of patient care. It is regarded as one of the most significant online resources for electronic health records, making it easier to send patient data from home to a doctor or other healthcare provider.

Due to some population, variables such as population increase policies are being taken that lead to reduced reliance on health care in the hospital, thus the patient becomes involved in this care as he plays an important role in making your health care decision.

Sometimes web services may be used by self-diagnosis Of the patient in particular cases and this, in turn, leads to determine whether the patient needs to be consulted by a clinical specialist or not.

Apart from the aforementioned benefits, the availability of these services helps the patient and the physician. The patient can identify healthy lifestyle choices and self-care practices, read about them, and reap their benefits, while the physician utilizes these websites to search for medical information and to participate in it. It should be noted that the purpose of websites is to provide general information about the patient, including some of the health issues they may be facing. This allows the patient to search for information at any time, and examples of these issues include quitting smoking and obesity causes.

- **Electronic Health or Medical Records (EHR, EMR)—General Overview**

One of the most crucial components of the hospital information system is the health record. They read medical records and make medical information easier to access. Additionally, it makes it simple for users to access and search for information. The terms computer-based patient records (CPR), computerized medical records (CMR), patient-carried medical records (PMR), electronic patient records (EPR), electronic medical records (EMR), personal health records (PHR), and digital medical records (DMR) are just a few of the terms used in the trade of electronic records.

The collection of health information about paperwork is different from electronic health care, so that by using the files and folders, the collection of information becomes difficult, as information is collected for the patient at each visit. Otherwise, the health information is collected once and returned to it at any time.

We observe that employees in the health sector bear a heavy burden when it comes to gathering data and medical records from patients who use paper records, and that when electronic records are used, patients are more likely to participate in the information gathering process, which raises the standard of care. The process of using electronic records involves converting paper records into electronic data that contains patient information, physician observations, prescription information, and any necessary analysis.Patients' records are treated by the hospital staff as a store that contains all the basic and necessary information in all types of primary, secondary and tertiary care, where it is used for the purposes of the most important of which is to facilitate patient service, data preservation and evaluation of its results.

In theory, patients can obtain patient data more easily and at any time by using the e-care system. In a similar vein, the doctor has profited from this service since it allows him to see a greater number of patients than he would if he worked within the confines of a medical facility.

The process of gathering patient data from the clinic used to be a little challenging because the nurse had to search through papers and documents, use a fax machine, or call someone. Fortunately, the use of electronic records made their job easier because they could access the necessary data whenever they needed it.

A number of outpatient primary care clinics have adopted the use of an electronic health record system in their practices.

Recently in the most developed countries, the electronic health record is adopted significantly. It is adopted as an important application in the field of health care by providing electronic patient records and these are considered as the most important electronic health care services.

Many developed countries support the electronic registry system as well as national health records and through huge investments in this field.

• **Telehealth or Telemedicine**

The use of an IT system to deliver health services remotely is known as telemedicine. This is done when the doctor and patient are not in the same location—that is, when the patient is in a distant location and the doctor is in a different location. Telemedicine comes in two flavors: the basic kind, which is done over the phone to address issues, and the more complicated kind that uses satellite technology. The quick advancement of technology has contributed to the rise of many people who are unable to obtain healthcare directly from special centers, which is one of the primary causes of the emergence of this kind of tool.

It was previously difficult to allow the patient to participate in the doctor's self-monitoring of his health but after the use of telemedicine, which enabled many patients to educate and follow up their disease remotely and thus facilitate the health care of a large number of individuals.

As for the eternal health of the concurrent be through a visual connection using the phone and a dialogue between the doctor and the patient and discuss the health situation and here is delegated patient participation in the case, As for the secondary non-synchronous health comes the importance of non-transfer of data at regular intervals, which leads to the possibility of changing the results since the sender and the future should not be synchronized length of time, for example, when following a specific disease such as liver disease, the patient can access his data and follow-up treatment progress and this gives him Psychological condition is good.

• **M-Health**

Mobile health can be defined as the direct use of electronic devices for voice communication and the transfer of essential data from healthcare centers. Because information technology is developing so quickly, there has been a recent increase in the use of this kind of technology. The majority of member states use M-Health initiatives, according to a survey conducted by WHO and distributed to its member states. Of the 112 member states that responded, 83% said that their nation had at least one M-Health initiative.

In many hospitals, mobile phone usage is widely observed and with the increasing sophistication of information technology, this will lead to the adoption of mobile phone usage in the future.

Due to the rapid development of the health sector, wireless infrastructure has become a major and prominent role in most mobile communities.

• Mobile Phones

When it comes to tools, one of the most used pieces of technology worldwide is the phone. Physicians continued to treat patients over the phone and to advise it. The mobile phone's technological advancements have allowed patients and doctors to communicate instead of meeting in person or speaking at the same time. Serving the patient's medical needs in this way is simple. Because of the increasing sophistication of technology and its availability to consumers, the use of mobile phones has become important in providing health care services. The concept of health care is changed from one period to the next but it is expected that the health advice will be via mobile phone, most notably.

Methodology

This study set out to determine the effects of using the IT system in Yemeni hospitals and how, from the perspective of the hospital staff, it can enhance the delivery of healthcare. In order to accomplish this, the researcher employed the applied method in conjunction with the analytical descriptive method, which involved the use of various statistical techniques and treatments pertinent to the subject's study, all without the researcher's involvement. The researcher can therefore engage with these circumstances, examine and characterize them. The current study is an applied study based on descriptive analytical methodology using a questionnaire prepared by the researcher to be a tool to obtain the information needed by the applied side of the study and based on the available literature and related studies.

The study concludes a basic type of data, which is the primary data obtained from a systematic questionnaire distributed among health workers in Yemeni hospitals where the researcher tried to describe and analyze their views. After the distribution of the questionnaire and the collection of data, a statistical analysis was carried out in order to obtain the final report and the necessary results through a statistical program called SPSS.

Government and private hospitals were the two types used in the research. It is noteworthy that the proportion of public and private hospitals is comparatively near to one another. There were 207 government hospitals and 200 private hospitals among the respondents. This can be clarified by the finding that hospitals in the private sector account for nearly half of all human cadres. This could be because the researcher believes that the private sector is always growing because of its superior services, which draw a lot of patients and provide a significant financial boost to the hospital, leading to an increase in employment.

When explaining this point we note that the highest percentage of those who believe that the use of the IT system has positive effects and these positive effects, as they say, lies in that some patients when visiting a hospital in order to treat certain health problems, the patient should do all the Routine medical transactions that he has done every time. This, in turn, is difficult to work on the employee and also on the doctor because of the lack of a satisfactory history of the patient who may help the doctor to diagnose the situation better. And this, in turn, leads to the loss of some important information that helps in diagnosis; in addition, it becomes more expensive for the patient in each visit. This indicates that a high proportion of respondents aspire to the availability of the information technology system in the health care sector because of its positive effects to improve the health care services provided. This is shown in the table where the lowest percentage of respondents who expect the negative effects of using the information technology system.

Standards in Health Informatics

The sharing and exchange of information between departments, health agencies, and healthcare professionals is made possible through standards. They are required for the language, databases, system architectures, and information content in order to enable linkages between systems through an apparently seamless integration of widely dispersed systems. This is frequently denoted as "interoperability." Standards are necessary for electronic medical or health records in order to quickly retrieve health-related information through indexing and cataloging, as well as to collect consistent clinical data for research. Without standards, classification and coding systems we are unable to compare the health status, processes of health care, costs and outcomes between various treatment options, health agencies, regions or countries in a meaningful way. In industry generally the adoption of standards has resulted in an increase in market opportunities and lower costs for equipment and services to users. In health informatics the widespread adoption of standards is expected to improve the health of the nation's population at a lower cost by improving the ability of health professionals, public and health service administrators to share and make better use of the information generated.

Standards

A standard is a prescribed set of guidelines, conditions, or requirements that address things like term definitions, component classification, material specifications, operation performance, procedure delineation, or quantity and quality measurement when describing materials, products, systems, services, or practices. Benchmarks are standards. Effective standards are required to set technical requirements for data exchange via electronic means and to govern data access and usage conditions. This is necessary for accurate and economical data collection and storage, which improves the retrieval of high-quality health information required to get the right knowledge to support decisions. Information exchange requires standards which provide a mutual understanding of the meaning of the data used. That is a standard language is needed and the context within which health data are collected or other related information, such as a personal identifier, date and time which are related to clinical observations, must not be lost. Standards may be mandated or be adopted voluntarily. According to Megargle the quality of the knowledge thus obtained is dependent upon three factors, reliability, relevancy and responsiveness. This can only be delivered when standards dealing with for example electronic compatibility, characterencoding and message structuring, are adhered to by the many different computer environments and software programs which may need to be connected to make for example one hospital network. Standards development for health informatics requires input from discipline experts, that is those who need to use the information and knowledge provided by a system. Much of this knowledge now resides in medical records and the health related literature. Who develops standards? Various health and related professional groups, public and private organisations have established standards for paper based health records, for health information systems, for health service delivery and for the health professions. Many such organisations have also implemented mechanisms by which compliance with these standards could be measured. As the automation of health information and communication technology is progressing it has become more apparent that standards for documentation and electronic data interchange within the healthcare sector are urgently required if we are to maximise the benefits offered through the use of these new information and communication technologies. The health care sector has special communication needs. Several organisations nationally and internationally are addressing this issue from various perspectives. Many standards applicable to information and communication technology generally need to be adopted within the healthcare sector. But additional standards are required specifically to meet the unique needs of the health care sector especially in the areas of data specifications, data integrity and security. Increasingly these are being developed through the well established standards organisations such as Standards Australia, the European Standardisation Committee (CEN), the Institute of Electrical and Electronics Engineers (IEEE), the American Society for Testing Materials (ASTM), the American National Standards Institute (ANSI), the European Strategic Program for Research and Development in Information Technologies (ESPRIT), the International Standards Organisation (ISO), and many others or through ad hoc groups such as health level 7 (HL7). In 1991 Mandil noted that 'despite progress in recent years, the lack of standards remains a major impediment to technical and international collaboration in health and health informatics'. He went on to say that standards 'tend to liberate cornered clients but (that) they also increase uses of the technology and hence its clientele'. European standardisation activities for health informatics began in 1990 when the CEN established Technical Committee 251. Standards Australia established its IT/14 committee on health informatics early in 1991. A Healthcare Informatics Standards Planning Panel (HISPP) was established by ANSI late 1991 to bring together the many standards groups which had been developing medical informatics for nearly a decade. Since then many more activities have taken place. In 1993 CEN's Technical Committee 251 published a directory of the European standardisation requirements for health care informatics which includes a program for the development of standards. Also in 1993 CEN TC251 and ANSI/HISPP produced a publication detailing the worldwide progress made in standardisation in healthcare informatics (De Moor, McDonald, Noothoven van Goor 1993). Significant cooperation exists amongst the different standards organizations. Priorities for standard development are determined by factors such as economic impact, medical benefits, user requirements, and feasibility.

Standards should be developed

Every day, new government policies aimed at increasing accountability and controlling costs are being introduced, along with initiatives like the Advanced Informatics in Medicine (AIM) project, the Health Care Information and Communication Network (RICHE) in Europe, the Australian Health Communication Network (HCN), the development of systems to support electronic health records, and the creation of systems to support these initiatives. There is consensus that ultimately we will need longitudinal (from birth to death) electronic health records to overcome the problems and costs associated with a highly mobile population, increasing specialisation within the health sector, duplication of data collection, incomplete and inaccurate medical histories, incomplete data for research and policy development purposes. Three years ago Murphy reported that a standard description for the content and structure of an automated longitudinal health record was under development. European countries and the United States of America have allocated millions towards standards development in recognition of this need. It is postulated that accurate and complete information will lead to improved knowledge, better decision making, improved quality of care, less cost and better use of available resources. Gabrielli identified three reasons for why the medical record was slow to be automated. The first is because of the extensive use of narrative text, secondly because of a lack of a standard medical terminology and thirdly the lack of a medically useful taxonomic code scheme. As a result he notes that clinical experiences are available to others only via expensive research studies, manual monitoring of the quality of care is labour intensive, and health care policies are more intuitive than fact driven.

Adoption of standards

Standards adoption could be required or optional. There are several kinds of standards. This depends on who created or embraced the standard, as well as why it was created in the first place. For instance, a lot of efforts are focused on creating a common language in the medical field, which is covered in the previous chapter. There are three types of standards: industry standards, which are used by an entire industry, government standards like GOSIP (Government Open Systems Interconnection Profile), and consensus standards. Corporate standards are created and utilized by a single company. The latter are the result of input from all stakeholders and are the most useful but may take years to develop. The adoption of standards is achieved more rapidly when users or potential users insist that suppliers comply with consensus standards. One of the reasons the health care industry in Australia and possible other countries, is so far behind other industries in this regard is because purchasers have continued to acquire proprietry systems. As these vendors are unable to satisfy all health information needs, there is a proliferation of disparate systems and an industry devoted to connecting them with taylor made solutions (interfaces). On the other hand a generic and ultimately more cost effective solution providing faster connectivity, is to adopt the what is referred to as the 'open' solution, which requires only minor adjustments to link machines. Open systems are those with which other systems can communicate via highly distributed systems. However the extent of such 'openess' appears to vary. Bakkeridentified five different meanings for the term. Open systems may be characterised by the possibility to communicate with other systems, extract data for external use, import data from external systems in the database, run the system on different hardware platforms or to extend an information system with modules from an other supplier. The latter is possible only if different suppliers produce identical modules. Bakker provided an analogy with cars. Both cars and health information systems are made up of many parts, however the engine meant for one car does not necessarily fit another. He notes that for some of the essential aspects of openess consensus of users and standardisation are indispensable. Another chapter discusses data communications in more detail.

Standards are needed specifically to make sure that, when it comes to system security, systems allow adherence to privacy and freedom of information laws and to prevent unauthorised access to data. This subject is covered in another chapter. Standards are also necessary for the user interface from the standpoint of the user. These are taking time to emerge. Because users in the health sector frequently need to access a variety of different computer applications, the goal is to enable users to quickly navigate and use any system with minimal training.

www.ingramcontent.com/pod-product-compliance
Lightning Source LLC
LaVergne TN
LVHW031242190726
843493LV00010B/2981